AF262992

ALSO BY QUEEN AFUA

Heal Thyself: For Health and Longevity

The City of Wellness: Restoring Your Health Through the Seven Kitchens of Consciousness

Sacred Woman: A Guide to Healing the Feminine Body, Mind and Spirit

Circles of Wellness: A Guide to Planting, Cultivating and Harvesting Wellness

Planet Heal: What would you do to heal planet Earth?

Impeccable Listening: 21-Day Meditation Guide to Restore Your Superpower

ALSO BY SUPANOVA SLOM

The Holistic Remedy

WEBSITES

Supanovaslom.com

Queenafua.com

SupaMegaFoods.com

MAN, HEAL THYSELF

MAN, HEAL THYSELF

THE WELLNESS WARRIOR'S GUIDE TO SELF-MASTERY IN 12 WEEKS AND BEYOND

SUPANOVA SLOM
& QUEEN AFUA

ONE WORLD NEW YORK

This book is intended as a reference volume only, not as a medical text. The information provided herein is designed to help you make informed decisions about your wellness. It is not intended to be a substitute for any treatment that may have been prescribed by your doctor. It is sold with the understanding that neither the author nor the publisher is engaged in rendering medical advice. If you have a medical problem, we urge you to seek competent medical help from a qualified physician.

One World
An imprint of Random House
A division of Penguin Random House LLC
1745 Broadway, New York, NY 10019
oneworldlit.com
penguinrandomhouse.com

2026 One World Trade Paperback Original

Earlier editions of this work were published in 2012 and 2021.

ISBN 9780593734254
Ebook ISBN 9780593734261

Printed in the United States of America

1st Printing

Book Team: • Managing editor: Allie Fox • Production manager: Katie Zilberman • Production editor: Mark Birkey

Book design by Mary A. Wirth

The authorized representative in the EU for product safety and compliance is Penguin Random House Ireland, Morrison Chambers, 32 Nassau Street, Dublin D02 YH68, Ireland. https://eu-contact.penguin.ie

DEDICATION

I dedicate this Expansion Edition Text to my late great step father Baaba Heru Ankh Ra Semahj Se Ptah, lovingly known as Baaba Heru Semahj "The Ankh Man." A Khemetic master teacher and Wellness Warrior Juggernaut.

DEDICATION

A NOBLE CALL TO MAN HEALING THYSELF

In the spirit of resilience and transformation, we present to you this sacred document, *Man, Heal Thyself: The Wellness Warrior's Guide to Self-Mastery in 12 Weeks and Beyond*. It is dedicated to all men who embark on the profound quest for self-healing. To those who carry the weight of pain, who yearn for restoration and renewal, we honor you. This is a tribute to those who have faced adversity, endured abuse, and strived to break the cycle of hurt. To those seeking change and metamorphosis in their lives, *Man, Heal Thyself: The Wellness Warrior's Guide to Self-Mastery in 12 Weeks and Beyond* is dedicated to you.

We extend our heartfelt dedication to the young men—the torchbearers of tomorrow—who are hungry for peace, completeness, and encouragement. You are not alone in your struggles; your journey is significant, and your pursuit of wholeness is noble. To the men with broken hearts, shattered dreams, and weary souls, we stand with you in your quest for healing.

To the mighty warriors who find strength and solace in their recovery, we dedicate this message of hope. You are on the path to becoming the Supreme Man of Optimal Wellness, and we urge you to persevere. Keep moving forward, for every step you take is a testament to your courage and spirit.

To those who feel lost in the labyrinth of life, this dedication is especially for you. Whether you find yourself in a place of confinement or navigating the trials of existence, know that mighty prayers of liberation surround you. Each moment is an opportunity for transformation, and the light of hope shines bright, even in the darkest hours.

We also acknowledge the men who are blessed with financial abundance and stability. Your journey is equally important, for wellness is not just a state of being but a shared experience that uplifts all. To the millions of men who have faced challenges and have risen from the ashes, we recognize your strength and resilience.

Finally, this dedication extends to the women—the mothers, grandmothers, wives, sisters, and beloved partners—who stand steadfastly in support, waiting and praying as the men embark on their journeys of healing. Women, your love and faith are the pillars that uphold the paths to recovery.

Together, let us celebrate the spirit of healing and transformation. As we dedicate *Man, Heal Thyself: The Wellness Warrior's Guide to Self-Mastery in 12 Weeks and Beyond* to all men, may you find the strength to embrace your journey, the courage to face your challenges, and the wisdom to heal. You are worthy of this journey, and your pursuit of wellness is a noble endeavor that inspires us all.

Wellness Warrior Salute!

EPIGRAPH

MAN HEAL THYSELF MASTER AFFIRMATION 1

Repeat three times daily. One time for the Mind. One time for the Body. One time for the Spirit.

Arrange for me the way
may I renew myself
may I become strong.
—THE PAPYRUS OF ANI

MAN HEAL THYSELF MASTER AFFIRMATION 2

Repeat once daily.

MAY I OPEN MY TWO EYES WHICH ARE BLIND.
MAY I STRETCH OUT MY FEET
WHICH ARE FASTENED TOGETHER.
MAY MY LEGS BE STRONG AND RAISE ME UP.
I KNOW MY HEART
I HAVE GAINED POWER OVER MY TWO FEET.
I HAVE GAINED THE POWER
TO DO WHAT PLEASETH MY SOUL.
MAY MY SOUL AND BODY
NOT BE IMPRISONED.
I RISE AND SHINE . . .
I AM POWERFUL. I AM MIGHTY.
I COME FORTH IN PEACE.
—THE PAPYRUS OF ANI

THE VISION

FOREWORD

By Queen Afua

It's Thursday, November 4, 2024, at 4:00 in the morning, awakened by my social activist holistic visionary self on behalf of Man Heal Thyself. Channeling through my inner vision is that Man Heal Thyself is going to reach the prisons where millions of our men, Black Men, are living through the modern-day Jim Crow–style free labor run by corporations. Man Heal Thyself is going to shift them out of their condition, starting with the renewal and never letting the mind return there again. Bob Marley said it best: *"Emancipate yourselves from mental slavery, none but ourselves can free our minds."*

Man Heal Thyself is going to wake up and catch the man on the brink of a stroke, an aneurysm, or a heart attack due to toxic living, and pull him up into his holistic healing.

Man Heal Thyself is going to stop an act of domestic violence in its tracks and so repair that broken soul, body, and heart, transforming that man from a man of rage, violence, and mental illness to a Man of Peace who loves on his wife and children rather than bringing harm.

Man Heal Thyself is going to reach the talented young Hip-Hop artists who unbeknownst got caught up in a dangling carrot situation of a bait-and-switch music deal and instead got sexually assaulted. Man Heal Thyself will help him to wash away his shame and put him on his path to recovery by taking hold of this expanded text and enrolling in the 12-Week Man Heal Thyself Rites of Passage. The men in healing will have arms wrapped around them and be supported by Minister of Wellness SupaNova Slom, accompanied by the Director of Man Heal Thyself, Halleluyah Walcott, and the 12 Wise Men, the Healing Juggernauts.

Man Heal Thyself is going to remove the missteps and the regrets, the darkness and the "It's too late" mindset.

Man Heal Thyself is going to turn back the hands of time and give man a second chance, a bridge over troubled water, a new day, a deliverance, a return home, a great opportunity, a way out, and a way through to higher ground.

Man Heal Thyself is going to birth the Righteous Goodness of man, where gun violence ceases—and the streets protect a community, not harm it.

Man Heal Thyself is the catalyst to return back home, our fathers, our sons, our nephews, our grandfathers, our lovers, our champions, our protectors moving our men to rise up out of the ashes, out of the mud, and thus break the cycle of DNA trauma. Our men through each Man Heal Thyself pylon will blossom as Wellness Warriors.

To the daughters who are fatherless, Man Heal Thyself is going to give you back your father whole and healed, giving you hope and the promise of a safe home where love supreme dwells. Daughters, don't you weep no more, hold "*The Vision,*" send him to enter into these Rites of Passage where the men teach the men how to be MEN. It's Our Culture, Our Way, Our Heritage. Our men will be trained up and developed by OUR MEN, who know the way and the way WILL BE MADE!

Man Heal Thyself as a way of life, health, and longevity. It is time to spread through the Diaspora throughout the world. This Is the Grand Reset. This is the time where Healed Women will attract Wellness Warriors and conceive Returning Ancestors who are born out of Healed Wombs of the Highest Frequency. Birthing a new civilization of MA'AT, balancing truth and harmony born to this new day.

This is the Reset where Black Men will be the example for ALL men. They will now take the lead and lead the way for a new Humanity of Well Men who no longer are trapped in a crisis, but instead radiate the Golden Age. Man Heal Thyself will chant as our ancestors gone by: *"Golden Are My Limbs, Blue My Lotus Crown and Emerald My Body"* (of vitality).

Man Heal Thyself will exude an example of a man standing in his healing. Men in tune with nature, in tune with Universal Law, are men who holistically regenerate themselves through the elemental activation and attunement of Air, Fire, Water, and Earth.

Man Heal Thyself is calling up the buried Sages, the Medicine Man, the Spiritual Giants.

This is a sacred calling for the Prayer Warriors and the Mystics to rise up in these times of Great Despair and Great Promise to wash over the Earth. May they remind man to purge away greed, domination, oppression, and manipulation through fasting and prayer. *"Let A New Earth Rise, Let Another World Be Born."* In the words of beloved author, historian, and pioneer-creator of Pan-African and Africana studies, Dr. John Henrik Clarke, *"Give the World a New Humanity."*

LIBERATION THROUGH WELLNESS

PREFACE

By Queen Afua

I am a Brooklynite. Born to two Civil Rights leaders, my parents were Ephraim Robinson, an entrepreneur, and Ida Robinson, a master homemaker. I was raised as a Brownstone Princess with my two older brothers Albert and James. We lived between Crown Heights and Bedford Stuyvesant, where yes, the trees grew in Brooklyn. Where children played outside and girls jumped double Dutch. Where music was celebrated . . . Jazz, Soul, R&B, Hip-Hop . . . Where African Cultural Schools emerged to help us to reclaim our African Minds. And where brothers rapped to pretty black girls with afros and press and curls.

In Brooklyn, I gave birth to my Holistic Healing Center in my parents' four-story brownstone, where the community came to Heal and to commune with one another in wellness. Mothers, daughters, sisters, friends young and old came as my team, and I administered colonics, massages, vegan food preparation workshops, and the 21-Day Detox and Wellness Consultations to thousands over the years. The MEN came for healing back then, usually because their wives and daughters came and sometimes on their own, seeking out wellness.

They came, Stevie Wonder the Musician, Doug E. Fresh the Personality, Eric Adams before he was the New York City Mayor, Ralph Carter of *Good Times*, Les Brown the Motivator, Noreaga of the CNN Crew, LeRoy Campbell the Artist, Bob Law and Imhotep Gary Bird, Masters of Talk Radio on WBLS, WWRL, and WBAI. Grammy Award–winner Erykah Badu brought Andre 3000 of OutKast and Common by the house for healing to get into the wellness mix. It was a time before Spike Lee's movie *Crooklyn*. It was BROOKLYN! Before gentrification, it was the BLACK community. Before Random House was in my neighborhood, there were street book vendors. And there was A&B Publishing on Atlantic Avenue, which published my first book four decades ago, a little green book called *Heal Thyself for Health & Longevity*.

It was Heaven and Hell that pushed us into wellness. Black folks held weekend-long health parties. Black folks endured year-round food deserts. Drug infestation in our neighborhoods propelled us to *Heal Ourselves*! Before the Holistic Heyday of Brooklyn, my beginnings of wellness were started in 1969 in Harlem on 125th Street and Seventh Avenue by four brothers. These four Freedom Fighters for Wellness pooled their resources and opened a holistic cultural center for higher learning one block away from the world famous Apollo Theatre. Guided by the teachings of our Nile Valley Ancestors—the original Healers of KMT, the Black Land, the Freedom Fighters for Wellness named the center AQUARIUS LEARNING CENTER. The vision of the four men has not only inspired my work to this day but has also empowered my son, SupaNova Slom, who from birth was destined to grow up and become a healer.

The 4 Black Men of healing and business and getting "The BAG" back then were: Dr. John E. Moore, a Master Herbalist; Kanya McGee, an Astrologer and Metaphysician; Lloyd Strayhorn, a Numerologist; and John Harris, a Naturopath and Radio Personality of WBLS. They painted on the walls of the center images of *our people and our greatness*. They filled the bookshelves with African holistic knowledge and offered workshops to empower the people with uplifting information. The major offshoot of the project was the continuation of the Black Power consciousness of the Civil Rights Movement. We, *The People* came from far and near, hungry for the knowledge of self, of healing, of herbs and natural medicine, of alchemy, and of our history, all available at AQUARIUS LEARNING CENTER. We purchased from Black merchants, bought books written by Black authors, and absorbed knowledge and wisdom from the ages.

Soon after AQUARIUS was thriving, the men opened a Juice Bar across the street, also on 125th Street. The community was introduced to detoxification and natural living through freshly prepared juice therapy and liquid elixirs. The 4 Black Men did not LET UP! With Sister Ruth Harris, a Black Woman with a flair for beauty and business, the 4 Black Men joined forces and sponsored a healing retreat in Upstate New York. This was the retreat that, as a teen, changed my life forever and led me into optimal wellness. I never looked back.

These 4 Black Men impacted our lives as a people in the midst of the Civil Rights Movement, the Black Power Explosion, the Holistic Wellness Movement, the Metaphysical Movement, and the Yoga Movement. The 4 Black Men were ahead of their time and right on time! These Holistic Freedom Fighters and Liberated Entrepreneurs, these Healers loved their community to Wellness. They did it all for *US*. Serving vegetarian foods and live juices, they hosted Roof-Top Holistic Healing Parties with music played by the best DJ's in Harlem. These 4 Black Men created a wellness model where success meant healing our community despite the challenges. It became a time of blessings in self-tuning for wellness.

On the A train from Brooklyn to Harlem, I didn't miss a beat, and the beat was in.

I found myself interacting in a sister-girl tribe of healers. There was Dianna Pharr, Astrologer; Dr. Roshan, Metaphysician; Camelie Malott, Theatre and Dance Professional; and me, a Holistic Wellness Coach. During this time, Dick Gregory came out with his book *Dick Gregory's Natural Diet for Folks Who Eat: Cooking with Mother Nature*. Our sister tribe read books such as this and continued working with Mother Nature in the effort to develop our multiple tools for self-care and wellness.

From their birth, I raised my children with all I learned on my path. On the wings of the 4 Healed Men, I raised in Wellness: Sherease, my heart, my daughter; Ali, my youngest to carry the Legacy; and SupaNova Slom, my eldest and the Co-Author of *Man, Heal Thyself*, who I am certain birthed the Spirit and Rise of the Wellness Warrior, which my sons branded and live by as their code to holistic sovereignty.

Trauma such as domestic violence occurs far too frequently in the lives of our men. Far too frequently our men face health crises such as prostate cancer and erectile dysfunction, debilitating high blood pressure, kidney failure, and diabetes that steals toes, sight, and spirit. Prisons are filled, slave-ship style, with millions of our men—our geniuses. A tragedy.

Wellness Warriors SupaNova Slom (Man Heal Thyself's Minister of Wellness) and Halleluyah Walcott (Man Heal Thyself's Program Director), along with the 12 Healing Juggernauts are continuing the energy of the Freedom Fighters who were the Wellness Warrios of the '60s era. Standing in the gap of hopelessness, these men actively seek to end traumas by liberation through Wellness. Man Heal Thyself is the Medicine, is the Hope, and is the Vision designed to restore our men to wellness. As it was with the 4 Wise Men in the '60s, so shall it be now; in the spirit of redemption and overcoming, Man Heal Thyself is front and center.

PURIFY OR DIE!

PREFACE

I have so much appreciation for this collaboration between my mother, Queen Afua, and myself, SupaNova, with writing a wellness book for Men, about Men, and in honor of Men.

My holistic wellness training about what to eat and how to take care of my body began from birth. As a child, my mother had me teach and conduct workshops in yoga and Tai Chi for her client's children. Later, when I was a teenager, my mother asked me to give words of encouragement to her teenage clients while she consulted with their parents. We were a mother-son wellness team. I was honored! So it made sense that when I became a young man, my mother asked me to continue to address my peers, who are known as "Generation X." I spoke to young men—our future—about their wellness future. I told them, "Wake up and be healed!"

I wrote the book *The Holistic Remedy* and co-authored this text, which is a call to my community and the new generation at large.

WAKE UP!!! IT IS A STATE OF EMERGENCY!!! WE ARE IN AN URGENT HEALTH CRISIS!!! OUR FAMILIES ARE DYING!! MY GENERATION OF MEN IS THE FIRST THAT MAY NOT OUTLIVE THEIR PARENTS!!

In 2010, we mourned the passing of hip-hop icon Guru. I

challenged all of his peers and fans to not let his death be in vain. There is no reason that Guru and so many others under forty-five years old should be passing away at the rate they are. Every MC, B-Boy, DJ, Graf Artist, college student, "brutha" on the corner, G, and hustler is personally suffering from or knows someone battling cancer, arthritis, diabetes, asthma, hypertension, obesity, and many other illnesses. Most of these illnesses are caused or worsened by the foods we eat.

Don't think for one minute that your aunties, big mamas, and parents are the only ones battling these sicknesses. African American and Latino communities lead the statistics for all of these crippling diseases. People under age forty are being hit at alarming rates. According to the Office of Minority Health, about four out of five African American women are overweight or obese. Over 30 percent of African American children are at high risk for high blood pressure, diabetes, high cholesterol, and a slew of other obesity-related diseases.

Fast food, along with the overprocessed, prepackaged US food culture, has driven us to this place. If we do not act soon, we may not be able to turn back. Beloved Brother, do you still think this urgent health crisis does not apply to you? Or perhaps are you in need of some extra reinforcement?

Read the list below of globally renowned male celebrities who have battled major life-threatening health conditions. This list represents sons and fathers—the men of our future.

Juice WRLD	dead at 21—drug overdose
Gaines Adams	dead at 26—cardiac arrest
Big Pun	dead at 28—heart attack
Bobby Brown Jr.	dead at 28—cause of death unreleased
Eazy-E	dead at 31—AIDS
J. Dilla	dead at 32—cardiac arrest

Chris "Mac Daddy" Kelly	dead at 34—drug overdose
Fred the Godson	dead at 35—complications related to coronavirus
Ol' Dirty Bastard	dead at 35—drug overdose
MC Breed	dead at 37—kidney failure
Nate Dogg	dead at 41—stroke
Prodigy	dead at 42—complications related to sickle cell anemia
Thomas Mikal Ford	dead at 42—ruptured abdominal aneurysm
Chadwick Boseman	dead at 43—colon cancer
Heavy D	dead at 44—stroke
Phife Dawg	dead at 45—complications related to type 1 diabetes and kidney transplant
Craig Mack	dead at 47—heart failure
Anthony Mason	dead at 48—heart attack
MF Doom	dead at 49—cause of death unreleased
John Singleton	dead at 51—stroke
Kristoff St. John	dead at 52—hypertrophic heart failure
Michael Clarke Duncan	dead at 54—respiratory failure, heart attack 2 months prior to his death
John "Ecstasy" Fletcher	dead at 56—cause of death unreleased
Prince	dead at 57—drug overdose
Big Bang Hank	dead at 58—cancer
Andre Harrell	dead at 59—heart failure
Tommy "Tiny" Lister	dead at 62—complications related to coronavirus

Alonzo Mourning	kidney transplant at 33
Ghostface Killah	diagnosed with type 1 diabetes at 26
Boosie Badazz (formerly Lil Boosie)	diagnosed with type 1 diabetes at 26; takes insulin 3 times a day
Dr. Dre	aneurysm at 55
Irv Gotti	dead at 54—stroke, diabetes
Sacha Jenkins	dead at 43—complications from multiple system atrophy
Young Noble	dead at 47—self-inflicted gunshot wound
Biz Markie	dead at 57—diabetes complications
Rich Homie Quan	dead at 34—drug overdose
Coolio	dead at 59—drug overdose
Shock G	dead at 57—accidental overdose
Bushwick Bill	dead at 52—pancreatic cancer
DJ Mister Cee	dead at 57—complications from diabetes
Magoo	dead at 50—heart attack
Fatman Scoop	dead at 53—cardiovascular disease
DJ Clark Kent	dead at 58—colon cancer

Even though the celebrities listed above do not lack money, they still fall sick with disease because they have limited knowledge of how to "Heal Thyself." Dear Brother, you don't have to be old, poor, overweight, or living in the hood to be sick. We suffer from lack of knowledge. This microcosmic list is an example of what is taking place with our men on a macrocosmic level.

Beyond being a hip-hop artist, I am a second-generation

holistic health advocate. I have traveled the road with Grammy Award–winner, hip-hop singer and songwriter Erykah Badu as her wellness coach. Over the years, I have encountered countless celebrities dealing with minor and major ailments. On the personal front, I am sick and tired of losing young people and reading depressing statistics. At this point NOBODY IS EXEMPT. Everyone is vulnerable to these diseases, and unless we make some immediate major changes to incorporate healthier eating habits and lifestyle practices, my generation might not live to see fifty years old.

Dear Brother, if you are living on the American diet, YOU TOO ARE A WALKING, TICKING TIME BOMB, ready to explode at any moment from the buildup of fast food, fried foods, candy, sodas, sugary drinks, and chemical additives that you are constantly ingesting. I am talking to YOU.

In her book *City of Wellness,* my mother, Queen Afua, writes about fast-food corporate kitchens. Most people know that this kind of food is bad for them, but they continue to eat this way every single day. So I ask everyone, at what point are we going to WAKE UP?!!! The number one excuse people give for unhealthy eating is that eating healthily costs too much. Yet, many of these same people spend hundreds of dollars on expensive, so-called luxury sneakers, handbags, car rims, and other material indulgences. When we tell these same people who may buy two or three bottles in the club to go buy a juicer, they say it is too expensive or they simply laugh it off. Our priorities are horribly messed up when it comes to spending money and taking care of ourselves. People care more about what they look like on the outside than they do about how their bodies are working on the inside. They are more concerned with being able to participate in the "Pass the . . . / Blame it on the Alcohol" lifestyle than learning to do away with the sicknesses that force them to take medication daily.

They would rather invest in expensive shoes than work to prevent the diabetes that could one day lead to amputations and no more ability to wear shoes.

Big Pun passed. We didn't take heed. Nate Dogg had two strokes and passed. Not much was said. When we lost J. Dilla, people finally started to show some concern. When Phife Dawg exposed his battle with diabetes, which ultimately caused his untimely death, people began to realize that there was an issue. Still, no one has effectively challenged our generation on a widespread scale to reclaim our wellness at every level.

I challenge men to "Man Up" and "Heal Thyself" as we guide you through the Journey to Self-Mastery. I challenge you to lead a lifestyle not of disease that will continue to disable you but rather of wellness that will holistically empower your life as a Man.

SupaNova Slom

RECORDING ARTIST

PUBLISHED AUTHOR

HOLISTIC WELLNESS WARRIOR

CONTENTS

INTRODUCTION

My journey into wellness began long before I actually understood what it meant to heal thyself. For our family, the "Heal Thyself" concept began with my mother. Growing up, my mother's poor health issues caused her to seek medical solutions to her daily ailments. She was repeatedly told, "We can't help you." Finally, she met master holistic healers who taught her detoxing and fasting and other holistic practices. Proactively, she adopted a holistic lifestyle. My mother was on a mission to achieve her wellness. Over the years, she became the wellness guru known as Queen Afua. She was a beacon of holistic health who deeply believed in the power of liberation through purification, nature, nutrition, and spiritual wellness. She was consulted by clients and advised them that self-care and self-mastery are crucial for everyone's well-being. With perseverance, Queen opened her first Heal Thyself center in 1982.

It followed that when Queen Afua became a mother she would teach her children the value of holistic health. From my birth (in 1977) through the births of my brother and sister, my mother steeped us in the belief that with the right self-care, the body would always find its way back to balance. This act of balance, self-accountability, and self-love paves the way for true transformation. Self-care and self-mastery are crucial for everyone's well-being.

Our home was filled with the soothing aromatherapy of

essential oils. We drank herbal teas, cleansing detox drinks, and fresh green juices that I watched her make. My mother emphasized that food was medicine and raised my siblings and me as plant-based vegans (then called vegetarians), an oddity rejected by our extended family circle. In the 1980s and 1990s, holistic lifestyle was usually stigmatized and ostracized by the mainstream community. Nonetheless, Mom counseled her clients and instilled in her children the same principles. She steadfastly insisted that the greatest investment one can make is to nourish self through meditation, exercise, nutrition, and setting intention. I witnessed firsthand the resilience it took for her to prioritize holistic well-being in an environment frequently resistant to this *different* way of living. I was watching my mother be a warrior for wellness.

Observing wellness practices in our home and at the center, I learned meditation, yoga, Tai Chi, and even vegan food preparation. I must admit that at the time I was also an avid collector of G.I. Joe and Transformers toys. Assisting my mom by delivering products to her clients, I was able to earn *pocket change.* Pocket change was not enough. I asked my mother for more money to buy more toys. "More money means more responsibilities," she told me. "You *could* teach the children of my clients." So at the age of ten years old, every Saturday I taught forty-plus of my peers. Doing my best, I mirrored teaching some of the holistic practices my mother and her associates were teaching the parents. It worked. I earned more than pocket change, and I could buy more toys for my collection. Meanwhile, as I absorbed these strong wellness foundations of self-care and positive determination, a shadow loomed over our family—my father's struggle with crack cocaine addiction.

My father, who was one of the top respiratory therapists in NYC, also believed in the healing arts of holistic wellness. He was a trained swordsman and held high honors in various martial arts disciplines. My father's addiction began after a series of devastating events: the divorce from my mother, the death of both his parents within one year, and the loss of his best friend, my uncle Charles, who had been diagnosed with HIV/AIDS, the plague of the day. These back-to-back tragedies led my father down a path of despair. Despite the heavy shadow of my father's addiction, my mother never gave up on his healing. Inspired by her unwavering belief in wellness, my brother and I tried to heal our father by serving him green drinks and detox tonics, hoping that the love and care we poured into these remedies might reach him where words could not.

To our amazement, something incredible began to happen—my father started requesting the drinks himself. "Son, where are those healing drinks? Make sure you bring me some of your mother's tonics." Repeating the words I often said to him, he would remind me, "Remember, Son, purify or die." My father was smart enough to recognize the lifeline those words offered. Nonetheless, his recovery process was slow-going. Simultaneously, my own journey to wellness was being choked with life-threatening challenges. I was on a seesaw between "serving tonics" and "becoming a street kid."

The turbulent times of the eighties and nineties existed not only within our family but in our neighborhood as well. Brooklyn, New York, provided the dangers of a hard-knock life that was especially inviting to young brothers like me. Drawn to the streets, I thought that by becoming a street kid, I might bond with my father and perhaps snap him out of his stupor. I got involved with the gang Lo-Lifes. Our motto, "LO from head to toe," reflected an obsession with Polo gear. Although I stayed away from selling drugs because of my father's addiction, I did become a young gun runner—a path that nearly led to my demise. I remember once trying to impress my father with $15K and guns. For a moment, it sobered him up. He urged me to get out of the streets and focus on everything my mother was teaching me, but his advice went in one ear and out the other. On that seesaw between two worlds—my mother's life-rejuvenating teachings and the chaos of the streets—I could have died.

In warrior mode, fighting for her son's life, my mother decided to send me to live with family down south. Of course, I was expected to complete my last year of high school. The lessons I learned from my family, "Take care of yourself and do the right thing," became etched in my soul. I avoided the certain destruction of my life, which would have been inevitable had I remained in the gang population. I achieved my high school diploma. When I returned to Brooklyn one year later, I was a renewed young man. *"Wellness Warrior Salute, Mom, your decision saved my life!"*

Back home. Brooklyn, 1995. I looked around. Most of the "homies" I had grown up with were dead, in jail, or just . . . gone. . . . A few remaining Lo-Lifes had resituated themselves into the fashion and music industries. Meanwhile, I was seeing too many of the young people of my generation navigating gang violence and now health disparities. The total unwellness around me inspired me to become active in several ways. I began to teach the holistic principles I had been learning and doing all my life. Compelled by a universal call for unity, I created my grassroots organization, "Unify the Hood, Heal the Hood." From 1995 until 2010—before I entered military service—my organization enabled me to foster healing circles within the gang-afflicted communities I myself once inhabited. Further, we were able to broker hundreds of peace treaties among the street tribes throughout my city and across the United States. Eventually, "Unify the Hood, Heal the Hood" became a sanctuary for teenagers and young adults scarred by gang violence and plagued by health disorders. Wow, I had made it through the nineties and into the new millennium!

In fall 2011, I enlisted in the army via the infantry. Infantry are rigorously trained to be "disciplined, physically and mentally tough, trained and proficient in my warrior tasks and drills." We dutifully followed orders to serve and protect our country. We are often thanked for our service. But was each combatant enabled to be of service to himself? Enabled to embrace his own self-care and *heal thyself* on all levels? During my time in active duty, I talked with many comrades, some already grappling with post-traumatic stress disorder and the lingering wounds of war. I seized countless opportunities to share with them the power of the healing principles I had learned to use for my own self-care and resilience. I asked my battle buddies about their plans for healing from our conflict experiences. Most of them responded that caretakers "back home" would fix them or that they were "okay" and didn't need healing. I posed a thought experiment: "Imagine if we applied the warrior discipline of our military training to our personal physical, mental, emotional, and spiritual well-being?" I continued to share my lessons, my holistic work, and the importance of heeding guidance from those who love and care for us as we make the transformative journey from darkness to wellness. When I reflected on the impact of my challenges and my accomplishments, I realized that I had always been in training for active service—beginning with my age-mates, continuing in my community, and then sharing with my military comrades. *"Man Heal Thyself!"*

Twenty years after my return from down south, my father eventually sobered up. I'm proud to say that he remained drug-free for almost a decade before he passed away. *"Man Heal Thyself!"*

"Man Heal Thyself" is an urgent call to every man, transcending the barriers of race, religion, class, and sexual orientation. From an early age, many men have been conditioned to suppress their deepest thoughts and emotions, fearing that vulnerability equals weakness. Society has imposed upon them the idea that their sole purpose is to provide for others, often at the cost of neglecting their own emotional well-being and authentic self-expression. The lack of holistic balance and self-expression has left men trapped in toxic relationship cycles, marked by oppressive dominance, disrespect, and contempt toward themselves and humanity.

"Man Heal Thyself" serves as a warrior's chant, urging men to embark on a soulful journey toward self-discovery, self-mastery, and a universal brotherhood of man. By diligently cultivating their wellness disciplines and rituals, men can strengthen their accountability and create a collective force fighting for a higher quality of life. It implores men to awaken their personal power, embrace accountability, and restore balance to their lives and the world.

Currently, men find themselves frustrated, unable to express their authentic selves for fear of rejection by loved ones and society. Lack of expression, combined with unaddressed childhood and adulthood trauma, creates a dangerous state wherein men struggle to function effectively. "Man Heal Thyself" is a call for healing, urging men to reclaim their power, freedom, and authentic selves beyond the confines of their challenging environments. The time has come for men to activate their personal power, heal their wounds, and overcome the obstacles hindering their ultimate success. *Man, Heal Thyself: The Wellness Warrior's Guide to Self-Mastery in 12 Weeks and Beyond*, an expanded edition of *MAN, HEAL THYSELF*, aims to guide and inspire men on their transformative journey. By committing to daily disciplines and completing the 12-week optimum wellness protocol, men have the opportunity to become activated Wellness Warriors. The additional tools and resources provided in this book serve to strengthen their continuous pursuit of self-mastery.

On my own journey of self-healing, I delved deep within myself to face the shadows that once haunted me. I worked on harnessing and detoxing from the negative experiences of my former street life as I transitioned from an adolescent into a young man. I forgave both myself and my father for our perceived weaknesses in those times when we had lacked strength. I found solace in reconciling with my past. I am a man who is on a continuous healing journey. It is the yearning of my spirit to share this imperative message with the brotherhood of man so that we may serve our highest selves with utmost dedication. In doing so, we can continue with positive service to our women and our children, and contribute to the transformative works in this world. Let this expanded edition be an inspiration for you to grow beyond your limitations, dear Wellness Warriors.

> Dear Brother, this is my heartfelt prayer for you. May you have the strength to conquer your demons, to forgive, and ultimately to unleash your inherent power. It is the power to care for and love oneself, regardless of the circumstances and unfortunate situations we encounter. I salute your unwavering commitment. Remember, Dear Brother, that you are enough.

It is a blessing for me to share these lessons here with you, readers, in this newest edition of *Man, Heal Thyself: The Wellness Warrior's Guide to Self-Mastery in 12 Weeks and Beyond.*

Activate, Mighty Men.

Congratulations, Wellness Warrior!

SupaNova Slom

MISSION STATEMENT

May we, Man Heal Thyself Wellness Warriors, no longer be prisoners and casualties of life's war as we fervently seek our full liberation. Man Heal Thyself is a path and journey of inner freedom, a road map to Divinity. It is the road of emancipation sparked and healed by the original Man. Man Heal Thyself consciousness is ultimately an answer to planetary healing. The journey we take is liberating and the destination is freedom. The price for freedom may be high, but the price that one pays for being imprisoned and cut off from the very breath of life is even higher still.

If one expects to sort out freedom and move from a dead to a living existence, one must have the courage to be willing to sacrifice one's old, worn-out, ineffective self. The tapestry that we as Man Heal Thyself Wellness Warriors boldly make through the Aritu emerges and weaves itself into a Seneb Freedom Blanket—a patchwork quilt that we wrap ourselves into to re-create our destinies as self-healers and self-emancipators.

As we ascend and grow into a Man Heal Thyself Wellness Warrior, we will heal in numerous, unlimited dimensions by way of prayer, affirmations, visualizations, movement, purification rites, fasting, live food eating, altar work, holistic nutrition, and nature cures. Man Heal Thyself offers us the legacy of our most ancient traditions and legacy of power and healing through the Doorways of Illumination. As we ascend as a Man Heal Thyself Wellness Warrior, we will meet and greet our inner healer, who holds the keys to Heaven on Earth. Our state of consciousness will soar as we journey on to uproot and purge the deteriorated, dilapidated part of ourselves.

As an already healed man, we will be inspired to grow immeasurably. As healed men, we will go from being frightened, withdrawn men to courageous ones. We will go from a state of confusion to a state of serenity; from a distrusting state to a trusting state; from spiteful men to compassionate, loving men; from weak to empowered men; from unconscious men to wise men; from an insane mind to a right, divine mind; from restlessness to contentment; from a bored being to a creative soul; from suppressive to expressive men. We will rise from a deflated to an inspired state; from depressed to joyful men; from disease-infested to disease-free men; from dishonest to honest men; from a follower to a leader who is a free thinker; from a pessimist to an optimist; and like Lotus Men of Nefer Atum we will blossom.

As we, Man Heal Thyself, travel through each Arit wheel of power, we will finally reach our divine seat of Asar, the Great Father of wisdom, power, and healing. Now that we are on our divine seat of higher mind, body, and spirit, we are fully charged to be crowned by the Supreme Man of Self-Mastery "who has made an end of his failings." He will aid and guide men who will reach out to others that too are seeking Planetary Healing. Man Heal Thyself in the making, we come from the four directions of north, south, east, and west. We are constantly unfolding and reinventing ourselves through the many doorways into our Divine Body Temple. As awakened Wellness Warriors, we will overcome diseases of body, mind, spirit, and relationships, thereby causing freedom to erupt within. For after all, Man Heal Thyself, your destination is FREEDOM and your quest is LIBERATION!

WELCOME HOME!

MAN, HEAL THYSELF

CHAPTER 1

THE WOUNDED MAN

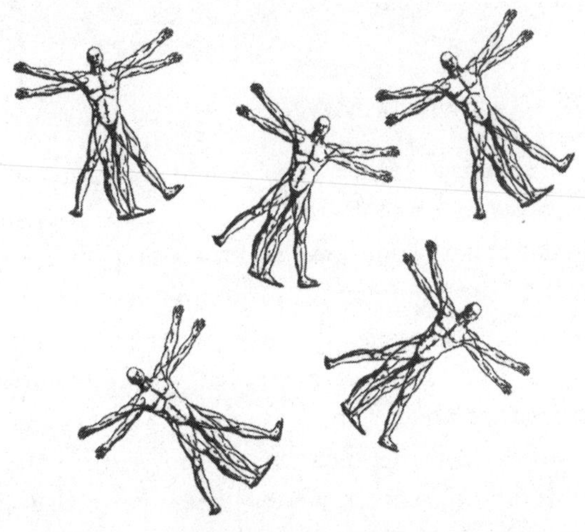

"Queen Afua made me aware that I could heal myself. . . . She was the first to talk to me about life with the solution being life."

—NOREAGA
Hip-Hop Artist

The reason a man would seek to heal himself is because in so many ways he has been wounded. This chapter takes a look at five types of men who are wounded in their physical, mental, spiritual, and social states of being. These wounds include the decline of man, the blockages in man, the issue of being "half a man," the attitudes of a man who lacks in many parts of his life. Men can overcome these states of *dis*ease. Once a man is honest with his emotions, then and only then can he transform himself into a natural, brilliant, loving, powerfully balanced man-state. He will be able to restore and secure his breath of life. Through the 12-week journey, he will learn how to restore and rejuvenate wellness to the 12 Aritu (checkpoints) so that eventually he can achieve optimal wellness socially, emotionally, and spiritually.

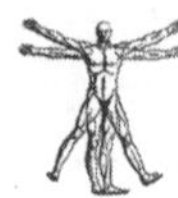

THE COMMON MAN

"Don't be common." Our mother would say this to my brothers and I whenever we, as children, "acted up." According to my mother, being "common" was the worst thing we could ever be. But "the Common Man" doesn't describe only those who are "acting up"; generally, he is a man who is normal and average. His life is complacent and uneventful; he lives safely in the bosom of mediocrity. A Common Man has Lack Syndrome, which keeps his life deficient, uneventful, and unfulfilled. A Common Man is a Wounded Man because his limited vision and low energy cause him to suffer from physical, emotional, social, sexual, and financial challenges. He is trapped in toxic, low-frequency, stressful, out-of-control relationships. A Common Man is disconnected from his inner and outer power mentally, physically, and spiritually. You must be willing to overcome the Common Man in order to Man Heal Thyself of Health and Longevity to the Supreme Man of Optimal Wellness.

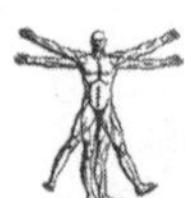

THE NEGATIVE ALPHA MAN

The phone rings. A man has called. He says, "*Queen, I heard your presentation in Atlanta, Georgia, at the Shrine of the Black Madonna. You spoke about the Negative Alpha Man. I felt you were talking about—and to—me.*" In a quivering voice, the man continues, "*I don't want to be that man any-*

more. I keep losing my mates because of the Negative Alpha Man influence, and I want to change. I have a mate at present, and I hope the Negative Alpha Man didn't already run her away like the others. It's like I can't control myself, like another me takes over. I start off as a Positive Alpha Man and then the moment I feel secure in the relationship the Negative Alpha Man kicks in, and I begin dominating and controlling the relationship. Queen, please help me, I want to be healed."

By the time Queen finished speaking with him, he was ready to claim his true self and take on the Wellness Warrior that would walk him through the 12 states of manhood. An Alpha Man in a negative state is a dominating, aggressive, pushy, short-fused, controlling, manipulating Know-It-All. He is verbally oppressive and abusive and maybe even physically violent. The Negative Alpha Man believes it's "his way or the highway." He's egotistically driven. The Negative Alpha Man does not share his full heart for fear of hurt, and he suppresses his problems and pain. The suppressed pain lashes out in a backhand slap to the woman, who, according to him, "talks too much." He hides himself in silence in hopes that no one finds out about his rage.

The Negative Alpha Man keeps his woman "in check" and under control and keeps her family and friends at a distance. The Negative Alpha Man views his mate as his property and wants to ensure that she is not influenced by what he views as "outside forces." The Negative Alpha Man has the skill to present himself as a Positive Alpha Man (page 12) to the public, but behind the door dwells the Negative Alpha Man. His wife is afraid, his children are distant, and his friends are concerned.

The Negative Alpha Man is emotionally unavailable to his wife after the honeymoon wears off. He pats his children on their heads, disciplines them, contributes to their upkeep; but don't expect him to rock, hold, or cradle them. After all, he provided the seed of them—that's enough, according to the Negative Alpha Man.

The Negative Alpha Man and the Positive Alpha Man do have one thing in common. Both believe that crying to release pain, hurt, and disappointment is a sign of weakness, when, in fact, if a man is able to cry when needed, he will be able to purify his heart. With the flow of his tears, his water element will become *un*dammed. This will cause his high blood pressure to lower and will prevent heart attacks and depression.

The Negative Alpha Man commonly works himself to death. Heart attacks and strokes are natural occurrences in the Negative Alpha Man. When a man treats his wife as his child and his children as his possessions, he is at the height of being the Negative Alpha Man. If, as a chronic Negative Alpha Man, you meet your reflection—a Negative Alpha Woman—and you want to save yourself, don't walk, RUN for your life onto the journey to Man Heal Thyself.

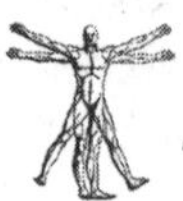

THE ANGRY OLD MAN

The Angry Old Man has a special chair that he sits in night after night. The chair has a dent in it because he's been sitting in it for so long. He sits his life away, watching television while other people win the game of life, or lose the girl, or fight for their beliefs. He lost control, and he can't seem to get out of the funk. He is stuck in the complacency that surrounds him. The Angry Old Man is a tired and depressed man that could be as young as 18 or as old as 88. An Angry Old Man is an attitude. The Angry Old Man is a man who has not fulfilled his life and whose dreams have been deferred. His hopes have not been realized, and his visions have yet to be manifested. As a result, the Angry Old Man feels empty of self-satisfaction and full of anger and regrets. He is angry because he has not been heard, he feels unappreciated, and he is not recognized for his gifts and talents. He is angry and old because his heart is filled with rage, hate, disgust, dismay, resentment, and hurt resulting from unhealed wounds of the past. He is angry and old because, unbeknownst to himself, he has created a box that he lives in with a sign on it that reads, "Stay Away! Love doesn't live here!" People around him get it, and they stay clear of the Angry Old Man. This only makes him angrier, for it's the aloneness that causes the anger to fester and results in the Angry Old Man harboring tension that keeps even the Angry Old Man away from himself—lacking self-love.

The Angry Old Man's state was planted in the sperm and in the ovum at the conception long before he was born and was passed down over generations. The Angry Old Man's state continued to grow when, as a small boy and as a youth, Daddy didn't hug him, or Mother ignored him, or both parents worked so hard that they didn't have much "lap time" to give him. Maybe he wasn't held as a baby at his mother's breast or in his father's arms; therefore, he suffers starvation for healthy touch. Perhaps he was a latchkey kid or lived in a single-parent home where he waited for Daddy, who never returned home. He might have experienced many false promises from the elders that were in fact broken, so as a youth, his heart shut down to protect him from more pain. He may have even been sexually assaulted, and so, as he carried his lack of love into his adulthood, the assault absolutely had to be a secret. The Angry Old Man runs away—from his children, his wife, his friends, himself. He seldom has anything good to speak on because he's so filled with what he feels—hurt turned into anger. The Angry Old Man could show up as demonic, for indeed what has happened is that the anger has turned in on itself and "possessed" the host.

The Angry Old Man has a special seat in his house that becomes his Throne of Anger. As a "couch potato," the Angry

Old Man sits and absorbs reflections of the pain in his own life while he stares at the lives of others—in pain—on the five and six and all-day and all-night o'clock news. He adds the bad news, sad news, violent news to his own pain, so the Angry Old Man's inner condition gets worse. The Angry Old Man ages quickly. His heart is weakened, broken, and heavy, and he is therefore a candidate for a sudden heart attack or slow-to-come stroke. For the Angry Old Man, the Common Man, and the Negative Alpha Man, there is a way out by bravely taking the journey through the 12 states of Man Heal Thyself to a Supreme Man of Optimal Living.

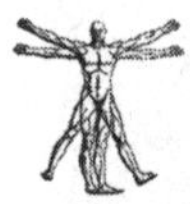

THE SEXUALLY ADDICTIVE MAN

The Sexually Addictive Man is possessed by a dark spirit that "rides" his mind, heart, and body. This spirit can possess the best and the rest of men. I witnessed some really powerful men who, as religious leaders, social justice leaders, cultural leaders, martial arts masters, presidents, CEOs, and artistic leaders, have succumbed to the sexually addictive spirit. In the news, we read and hear about these addictions as headline stories. I've witnessed men of nobility act as hustlers, pimps, sex fiends, and addicts with total disregard for their partner's body and/or emotions.

As the Sexually Addictive Man, an educated, intelligent, and otherwise "do-good" man gets so caught up that, even though he is more likely than not to get caught "out there with his pants down," he will give in to his addiction with sex. And he will do so anywhere—in a lavish four-star hotel or a rundown, at-the-end-of-town motel; in a truck or a tractor trailer at a highway rest stop; in the Oval Office; in a back alley; in his car; in the red-light district. Some men have sex night and day in cyberspace, empowered by a heavy diet of girly or manly magazines and videos. Even though he might get caught by his wife, his lover, his community, or his nation, the Sexually Addictive Man will take his chances because he is an addict. He can't say "No." He can't stop; he's out of control. He's got to get what he wants when he wants it; he just has to have it, regardless of the circumstances and consequences. These men will risk losing their children or damaging their reputation. Some sexually addicted men are sex offenders who hunt women or other men or children. Regardless of the circumstances, they will seek their prey to satisfy their addiction. Some addicts feel the need to have flesh-to-flesh touch so badly, they are willing to have sex without protection, which makes them automatically willing to spread viruses. Like playing Russian roulette with a loaded pistol to the head, they take their chances with their partner's life. With their irresponsible behavior, these perpetrators not only leave behind womb-war casualties (angry women), but they also acquire insurmountable karmic debt for which payment will be called, usually in the most unfortunate turn of events. Remember, for every action, there is an equal and opposite reaction. Some addicts have rotating girlfriends always keeping a warm vagina on standby. Some addicts set up a polygamy stable under the guise of cultural and religious righteousness. They have a different woman in bed with them Monday through Sunday. The woman not only performs sexual duties for him but also cooks, washes the dishes, cleans, does laundry, and performs childcare duties.

Some Sexually Addictive Men ejaculate so often that their sperm are weak and malnourished. This results in a debilitated brain, weak cells, and a challenged immune system. As the Sexually Addictive Man continues his destructive behavior toward others, he may suffer from impotence at an earlier age than expected. In addition, if the addicts are consumers of fried foods, junk food, and drugs, they become carriers of toxic sperm that poison their partner and produce dilapidated offspring.

Whether you were bottle-fed rather than breastfed or your father or your mother was not in the home or you were sexually abused as a child and beat up emotionally by women, men, lovers, partners, and mates, you can overcome the *dis*-ease of using your penis as an extension of your pain and a lethal weapon. Yes, you can heal. Man, take the walk of Man Heal Thyself and be whole. Stop passing your tension, your pollution, and your past misgivings onto your partner and calling it "sex" or "love" as you work out your inner disharmony inside your partner's body.

Men, save your life; elevate; raise your frequency; purge the hurt and *dis*ease from your body and your mind and your spirit. Be still as you restore peace and balance and control into your life. With each day of self-transformation, bear witness to a life of love rather than lust, peace rather than war.

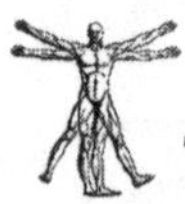

THE BROKEN MAN

A strong man came to Queen for consultation. His grandfather had just passed away. His grandfather had nurtured him throughout his life; they were close. His grandfather had been the root and the rock of the family. Upon his grandfather's transition into the spirit world, this young man's world fell apart. The women in his family broke down all around him, weeping and wailing. He was the only man left in his family. He was frightened of the responsibility of being in this position. As a trend, men do not outlive women; and this is unfortunately and certainly the norm in the African American community. In the average Black family, the men die between 45 to 65 years of age. The women live between 75 to 85 years of age. All the while, women are surviving hysterectomies, mastectomies, cancer, depression, and loneliness, all without men. Why is this?

Below are some of the conditions contributing to the early death of Black men in the United States. Statistics will vary, but these conditions also can be applied to men of African descent throughout the African Diaspora. In large numbers, Black men are suffering from heart attack, stroke, prostate cancer, and high blood pressure.

- 17.5% of the unemployed are Black men.
- 44% of the population in shelters are homeless Black men.
- 37% of Black men are obese.
- 72% of Black men come from single-parent homes.
- 36% of Black men are alcoholic.
- 33% of prisoners are Black men.
- 31% of gang activity exists in the urban community of the Black family.
- Unknown—the percentage of Black men who were sexually abused in their youth. The misplaced shame they harbor prevents them from sharing this tragic information. Therefore, the numbers are difficult to calculate, and the healing process is delayed or often never even begins. (Statistical data obtained from several sources. See Reference Section.)

I challenge the Broken Man to take the Journey to recapture, restore, reawaken yourself to wholeness. Give yourself daily wellness care so that you may live long and strong with your families. Overcome the Broken Man; instead become a Supreme Man of Self-Mastery and enjoy longevity as your reward.

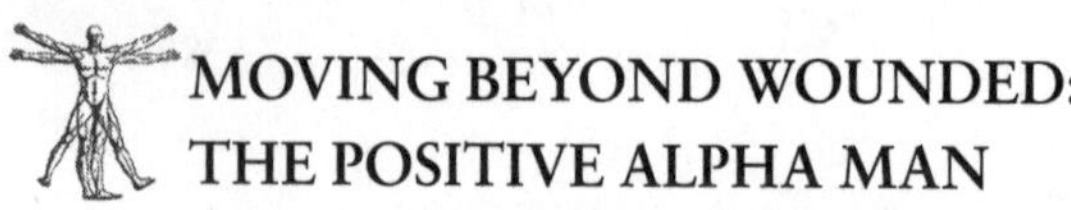

MOVING BEYOND WOUNDED: THE POSITIVE ALPHA MAN

A Positive Alpha Man is super powerful physically and mentally. He is strong-willed and determined to win in life despite challenges. A Positive Alpha Man is responsible and committed to whomever or whatever he believes in. The Positive Alpha Man takes care of his family, friends, and community. His parents are proud of him. His wife adores him, and his children openly love him. The Positive Alpha Man, who is in alignment with Divine Spirit, uses his blessing of unlimited creativity to ensure financial security for himself and his family. His friends respect him, and his community trusts in his profound wisdom.

You can always rely on the Positive Alpha Man to show up, to come through, and to make it happen. A Positive Alpha Man is dependable; he is "the Man." He has strong opinions. He speaks with authority, certainty, and intelligence and always assumes a leadership role. The Positive Alpha Man is well-read and spiritually in tune. He thinks outside the box. He is resourceful and knows that the power to manifest whatever he needs lies within. The Positive Alpha Man builds houses, bridges, families, hearts, and minds. He uplifts people and restores their lives. He is the backbone and muscle of any project. No matter what obstacles arise, he finds a way to get the job done.

Be advised that the Positive Alpha Man and the Negative Alpha Man have the same strength and energy. If the Positive Alpha Man falls off from living a positive lifestyle, he could become unfocused, and his ego could become compromised by challenges; he could flip-flop into the Negative Alpha Man. Therefore, Positive Alpha Man, be vigilant to practice holistic living daily so you can remain positive on the path leading to Self-Mastery.

CHAPTER **2**

THE HEALING POWER OF THE ELEMENTS

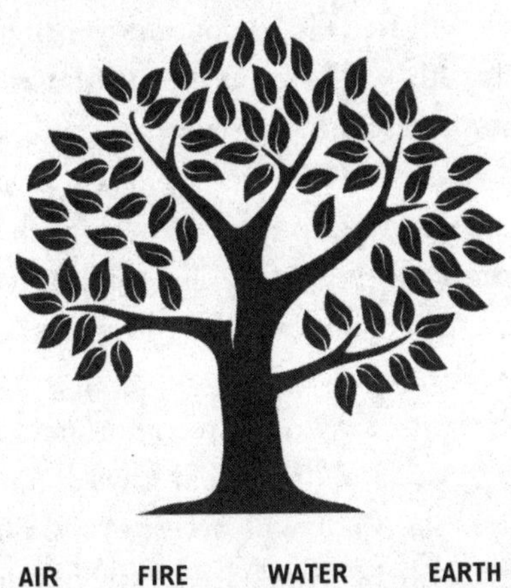

AIR FIRE WATER EARTH

"In the midst of the street of it, and on either side of the river, was there the tree of life, which bare twelve manner of fruits, and yielded her fruit every month: and the leaves of the tree were for the healing of the nations."

REVELATION 22:2 (KJV)

"We must sojourn on earth, to rediscover the light of our creation; we find that our passage is linked to the advancement of our issues of our earthly experience.

"We must discover what will bring to the highest potential for the cooperation of the elements that compose our body, mind, and soul. The elements of the earth sufficiently bring peace and stability within our cellular structure. By fasting and cleansing with the Man Heal Thyself regimen, we are prepared for life's journey."

—DR. PAUL BROWN BODHISE

author of *The Urban Sage: A Holistic Survival Kit for the New Millennium Truth Seeker*

THE JOURNEY TO THE 12 ARITU

Through the purification of one's anatomy for 12 weeks, a season of personal commitment to wellness, each man will reconstruct his body from limb to limb. Perhaps he will receive help from a wife, a friend, or a family member. Even better, maybe this man will be able to commit the time to take full responsibility for his wellness and Heal himself. He will be instructed on how to use the 12 Arit energy centers (also known as chakras), the use of affirmations directly from the temple walls of the Ancient African Ancestors from the Nile Valley, herbal compounds, fasting, Heal Thyself Lifestyle practices, clay treatments, inversion exercises, zone massages, green foods, wellness metaphysics, journaling, and the daily application of the elements: air, fire, water, and earth. Man will tap into his mighty power and thus, Heal Thyself.

Every 7 days, the man will activate another Arit, thus building from Arit 1–12. Awaken weekly, one inner conflict after the next. Each masculine aspect is addressed: from the Family Man, Sensual Man, Transformation Man, Lover Man, Communication Man, Intuitive Man, Universal Man, Illuminator Man, Harmonizer Man, Alchemist Man, to Supreme Man of Self-Mastery, fully aware!

To explore Man Heal Thyself, we will now delve into the elements to set the tone for aligning self to wellness with the air, fire, water, and earth tools of nature. Holistic empowerment shall restore Man to grace.

THE 4 ELEMENTS OF HEALING

Human Anatomy is a composite of 4 elements. The elements in the human body correspond with the 4 elements in nature: air, fire, water, and earth.

THE AIR ELEMENT: corresponds with the lungs/breathing.
THE FIRE ELEMENT: the Sun's rays—corresponds with the bloodstream and the reproductive organs.
THE WATER ELEMENTS: rivers, lakes, oceans—correspond to the bladder, circulatory system, and the kidneys.
THE EARTH ELEMENTS: the mountains and trees—correspond to the bones, joints, and colon.

The condition of a man's inner body is reflected in what he creates and in his relationship with himself, other people, and nature. The more vibrant and pure our inner elements are, the healthier and more harmonious our lives will be. The following information based on the elements will aid you in gaining a holistic life in body, mind, and spirit.

AIR ELEMENT

AIR THERAPY FOR OPTIMAL WELLNESS

Air rules the respiratory system. Breath is life. The quality of your life is determined by the velocity of the breath. The more active the oxygen flow of the breath, the greater the mental, physical, spiritual, and overall state of the body. We will gain healthier relationships that are more respectful and productive.

NEGATIVE SHALLOW BREATH

The breath has two opposing flows. One is a negative direction where the breath is constrictive, shallow, and weak. The negative breath disrupts tissues, cells, bones, muscles, and nerves. Negative breathing is due primarily to stress, emotional trauma, constipation, blockages of systems throughout the body, and/or a poor diet consisting of fast food, junk food, fried food. The negative breath creates the following negative conditions:

- Mental depression
- Shortness of breath
- Headaches
- Numbness in the hands, feet, and legs
- Impotence
- Poor memory
- Fatigue
- Lack of vision

HOW TO PERFORM THE POSITIVE BREATH

Sit on a comfortable chair. Align your head with your shoulders and your feet with your hips. Place your feet flat on the floor and your hands in your lap with palms facing upward. Align your mind with your heart and your heart with your body.

Inhale through your nostrils as you expand your lungs and abdomen. Exhale from your nostrils as you contract your abdomen and relax your lungs.

- Perform this breathing of 20 to 100 Lotus Fire Breaths 2 to 3 times a day. If you consciously practice the full-body breath, in time it will become your norm. With each breath, your body will be more enlivened.
- Over a season, increase to 1,000 Lotus Fire Breaths daily.
- Perform 250 Lotus Fire Breaths at each of these times: sunrise, midday, sunset, before bed.

MOVEMENT

Perform breathing exercises while performing yoga, Tai Chi, Ari Ankh Ka, dance, or power walking.

FORMULA: BREATH OF LIFE

For deeper, more vibrant breaths, take 2 or 3 drops of Heal Thyself Breath of Life formula with 8 to 16 ounces of distilled warm water and juice of a lemon.

THE RESULT OF POSITIVE VIBRANT BREATHING:

Positive breath flow is expansive, full, and strong. The positive breath brings oxygen to tissues, cells, bones, muscles, and nerves. Positive breathing will be the result of holistic eating habits, healthy relationships, and daily exercise.

FIRE ELEMENT

FIRE THERAPY FOR OPTIMAL WELLNESS

Fire rules the reproductive system, circulation, and the bloodstream. There is an Ancient Afrakan pose that is the grand master of all movements. The movement or pose is called "the Inversion." The Inversion Pose is to release the fire within to increase circulation throughout your anatomy.

POOR CIRCULATION

Man stands upright most of his life. As a result, as one matures, the energy and force travel down—away from the brain—causing poor memory; a clogged, weak heart; backache; prolapsed colon, bladder, and prostate; and swollen knees and ankles.

HOW TO PERFORM INVERSION FOR OPTIMAL CIRCULATION

ACTION

To perform inversion, you must lie flat on your back, preferably on the floor or on a bed, and place your feet against the wall at a 45-degree angle. This can be done on any flat surface where you can put your feet against a solid surface at an incline.

PREPARATION

Before inversion, mix equal parts olive oil and castor oil in a bowl. Apply this blend to your legs, arms, chest, abdomen, neck, and face. While in inversion, massage this oil blend vigorously into the aforementioned areas, concentrating on your organs—prostate, bladder, colon, and heart. Do this for a full 10 minutes to revitalize your body. Massage toward the heart for full revitalization effect:

- Better memory
- Strengthens heart
- Increases circulation
- Prevents prostate blockage and bladder disease

MOVEMENT

Soccer, basketball, kickboxing, martial arts, roller-skating. Perform 30 minutes to 1 hour daily.

THE RESULTS OF PERFORMING INVERSION

By inverting twice a day (every sunrise and sunset) for 10 to 15 minutes, man will increase blood circulation from the crown to the feet. Improved blood circulation will then help to improve memory; nourish the nervous system; strengthen the heart, bladder, colon, and prostate; and help to prevent numbing in feet and hands.

THE INVERSION AFFIRMATION FOR OPTIMAL CIRCULATION

You can combine the fire and breathing exercises for optimal benefits to the mind, body, and spirit. After doing the fire breath exercise (performed at sunrise and sunset), lie flat in the bed and place your legs against the wall at a 45-degree angle. Relax the body and inhale and exhale as you visualize that you are recharging each part of your body with the flow of life. Recite the following Ancient Inversion Healing Affirmation from the Nile Valley Ancestors.

- I am in the Utchat (Higher Consciousness, evolved mind)
  Nuk am ut'at

- I exist by its strength (My mind reflects my body)
  Au-a em maket-s

- I come forth, I shine (To go into meditation and come out vibrant)
  Aq-na aux a

- I have commanded my seat (I have power over my mind, my life)
  Atu-ma nest-a

- I maintain an exact balance (I am in harmony)
  Aqa- ua

- My form is inverted
  Ari-a sexet

- I open the door of Heaven (Balance)
  Ap sba em pet

- I am reborn on this day (Renewed)
  Nuk nesta em hru pen

WATER ELEMENT

WATER THERAPY FOR OPTIMAL WELLNESS

Water rules the circulatory system, bladder, and urinary tract. I know men usually prefer to take showers over taking baths. Showers are quick and easily done. Showers wash off the funk, clean the skin, freshen the soul. Man, to heal thyself, it is strongly recommended to bathe at least 3 times per week for

20 to 30 minutes. A bath can drain the toxicity from the body, and distress and anxiety from the mind. A bath rejuvenates the spirit. A bath can soften a cyst, break up plaque in the arteries, and prevent one from creating or attracting violence. Baths protect, support, and lift the body, mind, and spirit.

I offer 7 baths for you to use in order that your body can "drink" in wellness through the millions of pores in your skin. I also offer 6 tonics to be taken orally for flushing toxins from the body. The bath recommendations are as follows:

PREPARATION: BATH TONICS

Take 3 baths weekly; avoid salt and ginger baths if you suffer from high blood pressure.

1. **DEAD SEA SALT OR EPSOM SALT—TO DE-STRESS** (avoid this bath if you have high blood pressure)
   Add 1 to 2 pounds of bath salt to warm water. Bathe in the salt bath. Drink the herbal tonic that corresponds to the target organ or situation for which you are bathing.

2. **MASTER HERBAL BATH—TO DETOXIFY**
   Boil 4 cups of water. Turn off the flame and add 4 teaspoons of Master Herbal Formula to the water and steep 1 to 4 hours. Strain the herbs and pour the liquid into the tub. As a bath, use 3 times per week. As a tonic, drink 1 cup of Master Herbal Formula with 12 ounces of water throughout the day until finished. It can be used daily as a tonic.

3. **GARLIC BATH—TO LOWER PRESSURE**
   Remove 5 to 10 cloves from a garlic bulb. Blend with 4 ounces of water then pour into the tub. Add 1 or 2 drops of Queen Afua Breath of Life to the bath. You can drink this same solution of water, garlic, and Breath of Life.

4. **LEMON BATH—TO BREAK UP CONGESTION**
   Juice 5 lemons and add the juice to the bath. As a tonic, juice 1 lemon and add to 12 to 16 ounces of water and drink.

5. **GINGER BATH—TO IMPROVE CIRCULATION AND VITALITY**
   Juice ½ to 1 cup of ginger from fresh ginger root, then add to the bath. As a tonic, take 1 to 2 tablespoons of fresh ginger with 12 to 16 ounces of warm water and drink.

6. **ORGANIC APPLE CIDER VINEGAR BATH—TO BREAK UP CONGESTION**
   Add ½ to 1 cup of ACV to bathwater. As a tonic, add 1 to 2 tablespoons of ACV to 12 to 16 ounces of water and drink.

7. **BLADDERWRACK, FENNEL, AND CHICKWEED HERBS—TO REDUCE SWELLING IN LEGS, FACE, HANDS, ANKLES, AND KIDNEYS**
   Add 1 to 2 teaspoons of each herb to 1 quart of water. Steep overnight, strain, and pour into the tub. Reserve some of this tonic for you to drink as you bathe.

HOW TO USE THE WATER ELEMENT TO CLEANSE:

FORMULA

Take 3 to 4 teaspoons of the Queen Afua Master Herbal Formula to increase circulation.

ACTION

Take 2 to 4 salt baths 3 to 4 times a week. Use 1 to 2 pounds of Epsom or Dead Sea salt* or 1 cup apple cider vinegar. Take hot and cold showers daily.

---

* Use apple cider vinegar instead of salt if you have high blood pressure.

MOVEMENT

Rebounding, jumping, swimming, and massaging to move the lymphatic system. Perform 30 minutes to 1 hour daily.

EARTH ELEMENT

EARTH THERAPY FOR OPTIMAL WELLNESS

Earth rules the bones and colon. The 4 Element Green Living Program presents a systematic green-living way to restore one's anatomy on spiritual, emotional, and physical levels by using plants. Reach optimal wellness using a plant-based diet, daily ingesting up to 1 pint of a green drink. Create your green drink by adding 1 to 2 tablespoons of Queen Afua Nutritional Formula to green vegetable juice or water.

Drinking up to 1 pint of green juice drink daily for two weeks consecutively helps break the cycle of chronic disease.

The Heal Thyself Green Life Formula is a nutritionally sound compound that contains a full range of vitamins such as A, B complex, C, E, as well as bioflavonoids, choline, essential fatty acids, selenium, inositol, plus minerals such as calcium, copper, iodine, magnesium, manganese, phosphorus, silicon, sodium, sulfur, and zinc. Green Life also contains wheatgrass, a soil-based plant, and spirulina, a water-based plant that will rejuvenate and detoxify.

This intensive system of rejuvenation will aid in establishing a skeletal structure free of pain and a colon free of impacted waste to nourish your body and raise your frequency. Performing the suggested earth therapies also assists in overcoming rage, jealousy, verbal abuse, envy, selfishness, depression, procrastination, and the desire to perform destructive sexual activities.

HOW TO PERFORM EARTH THERAPY:

PREPARATION: FORMULA

Drink 2 to 3 (8-ounce) glasses of freshly pressed Green Juice with 1 tablespoon of Heal Thyself Green Life Nutritional Formula.

ACTION

Apply Queen Afua Rejuvenation Clay treatment to areas of pain 2 to 4 times a week.

MOVEMENT

Biking, jogging, power walking, calisthenics, weight lifting, or drumming. Perform 30 minutes to 1 hour daily.

RECITE

"May I be protected by 70 purifications. I purify myself at the great stream of the galaxy, and that which is wrong in me is pardoned, and the spots upon my body and upon the earth are washed away. I come that I may purify this soul of mine in the Most High Degree."

CHAPTER 3

ENTER THE WELLNESS WARRIOR

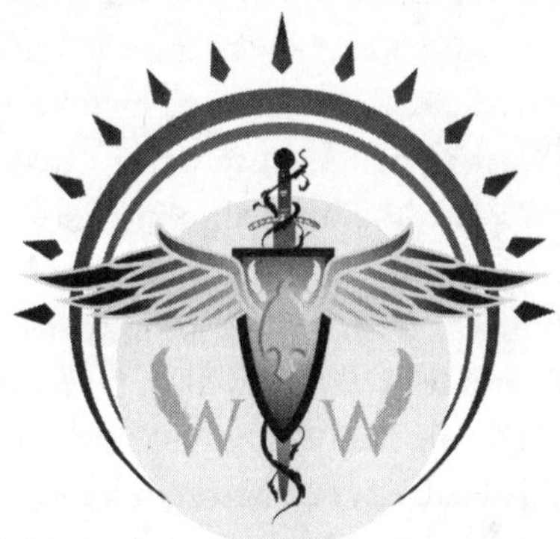

THE WELLNESS WARRIOR SHIELD

THE WELLNESS WARRIOR PROTECTIVE SHIELD CONTAINS:

The feather of Ma'at, symbol of balance, truth, and justice, and the sword of Bes, to move beyond your limitations by cutting away corruptible matter.

The Falcon is in the center to symbolize the king of the air, leadership, and self-mastery.

The circle depicts a continuum of eternal movement.

The Wellness Warrior Creed is simply "Purify or Die."

—SUPANOVA SLOM

THE WELLNESS WARRIOR MAN

We recognize and salute the Wellness Warrior Man and Healing Champion Man who have traveled beyond the state of the Common Man. You are the men on the Man Heal Thyself journey. You are still on the Quest to becoming Supreme Men of Self-Mastery.

The Wellness Warrior Man is diligent on his path to wellness. It takes your full force, your full attention, and your convictions to break the cycle of toxic mental, physical, sexual, and dietary addictions and tap into your inner wholeness. The Wellness Warrior Man has come to the awareness that to Heal Thyself, he must fight to receive and maintain his wellness. The Wellness Warrior fights to overcome a toxic lifestyle.

To maintain a healthy and vibrant lifestyle, the Wellness Warrior lives detoxification and rejuvenation techniques daily. He protects himself from falling prey to toxic living with drugs, alcohol, and tobacco, as well as flesh food, junk food, and microwaved food. The Wellness Warrior transforms himself by any means necessary to become enlightened and whole in body, mind, and spirit. The Wellness Warrior is a force to be reckoned with; he will fight for his wellness. His battle tools are determination, commitment, and conviction. The Wellness Warrior not only will defend his right to live a healthy vibrant life, he also fights for the wellness restoration and rejuvenation of his family, friends, associates, and community. He is a warrior for the global population's right to wellness.

Just as Bes (the Spiritual Guardian of Evolution and Transformation) takes the sword and cuts away corruptible matter and disease, the Wellness Warrior uses his spiritual sword to cut away issues and desires that diminish his life force. He will place the feather of Ma'at (balance and harmony) over the wounds as he transforms into the hawk and flies above all adversity to his Optimal Wellness.

I say to the Wellness Warrior Man with the conviction to be made whole, "Pick up your shield and sword as you cut away obstructions and continue your journey to defend wellness for yourself and others."

MAN HEAL THYSELF GLOBAL CIRCLE OF UNITY

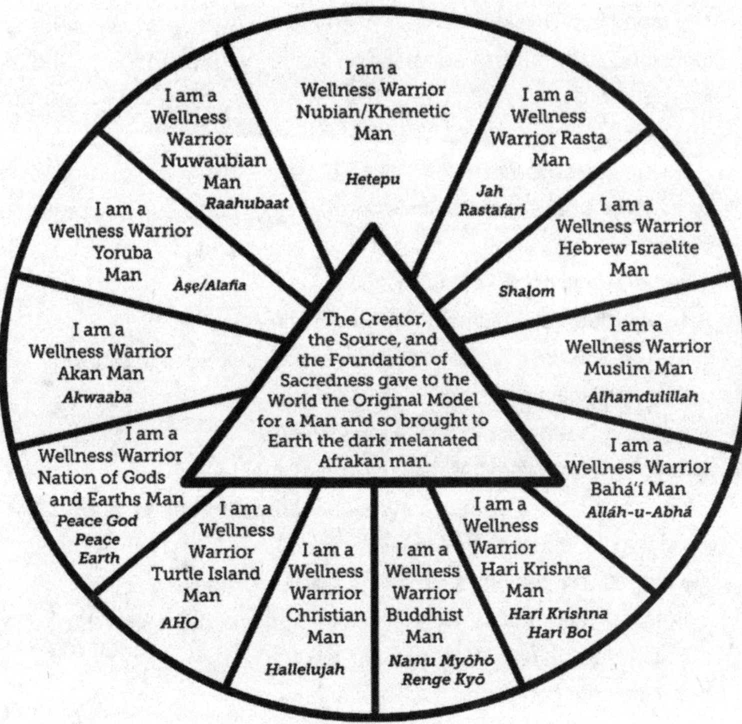

MAN HEAL THYSELF

WELLNESS WARRIOR OATH

The Man Heal Thyself Wellness Warrior Oath is a power charge to affirm your daily progress and journey toward Self-Mastery. Recite the Man Heal Thyself Wellness Warrior Oath every day as an empowering daily ritual to activate and sustain your mind, body, and spirit's wellness.

As a Wellness Warrior, each day I pledge
to honor the health and wellness of my mind, body, and spirit with
high-vibrational awareness of my choices and interactions,
whether within or outside of myself.
I make a deep commitment to my commitments
24/7 and 365 days of the year to defend myself against all toxic
foreign enemies that are outside of me,
such as viruses, people, places, and things.
I make a deep commitment to my commitments
24/7 and 365 days of the year to defend myself against all toxic
domestic enemies that are within me,
such as toxic thoughts, toxic habits, and blockages.
I protect myself against all enemies foreign and domestic as a
Man Heal Thyself Wellness Warrior
because I am committed to personal development
and transfiguration daily.
Every day is a new gift, a new opportunity, and a new chance
for a greater quality of life and for
Optimal Wellness through Self-Mastery!

WORD POWER!!! AFFIRM DAILY!!

MAN HEAL THYSELF

WELLNESS WARRIOR CREED

The Man Heal Thyself Wellness Warrior Creed is a power charge to affirm your daily progress and journey toward Self-Mastery. Recite the Man Heal Thyself Wellness Warrior Creed every day as an empowering daily ritual to activate and sustain your mind, body, and spirit's wellness.

Because I am a Wellness Warrior, no matter where I am deployed in life, I will honor my wellness.
As a Man Heal Thyself Wellness Warrior, no matter my job description
and no matter where I find myself on this planet, I make no excuses for honoring my wellness.
No matter the demands or chaos of life, my well-being is a priority.
I will not compromise the opportunity to build and to obtain
a greater quality of life for Self-Mastery!
NO EXCUSES, WELLNESS is my creed!

WORD POWER!!! AFFIRM DAILY!!

CHAPTER 4

MAN ON HIS HEALING WAY

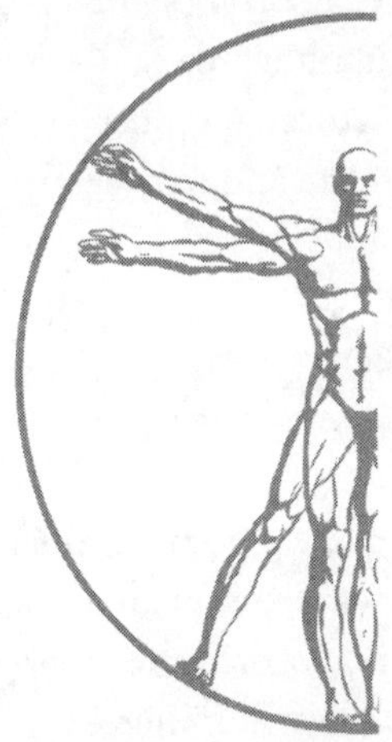

"Health is the most important thing this universe has. It is the first and last of your existence or existing.

A wise man has good health because of love for the body.

Love is injected and then projected.

Self-love shaped and shapes the universe."

—DR. PAUL GOSS
Author of *The Natural Way*
Founder of *New Body Products*

PREPARING FOR THE MAN HEAL THYSELF JOURNEY

PREPARE YOUR MIND.

Read material on wellness. Although your decision to detox is a private and individual one, for support you may choose to speak to others who are on the path to becoming a Supreme Man of Optimal Wellness.

PREPARE YOUR SPIRIT.

Consider reciting and reflecting upon the affirmations from both the Heal Thyself affirmations. The Teachings of Antiquity were based on the principles of Ma'at: Truth, Balance, Justice, and the Knowledge of oneself.

Choose and reflect upon words that are appropriate to the situation you want to restore to wellness, or the body part you are focusing on to revitalize and rejuvenate.

PREPARE FOR AND PERFORM MAN HEAL THYSELF MEDITATION AND VISION QUEST.

STEP 1

Early Morning Rise between 4 a.m. and 6 a.m. to maximize your soul's connection with your meditation and affirmations. Cleanse your internal body; drink 16 ounces of warm water with the juice of 1 to 2 lemons or limes.

STEP 2

Cleanse your spiritual channel; quiet your mind and spirit.

STEP 3

Recite Man Heal Thyself Healing and Harmonizing Meditation (Master Affirmations 1 and 2 in epigraph).

Sit on a comfortable seat with your back straight, shoulders down, chest open, and palms open. Close your eyes and go within your heart as you connect to your breath. Now inhale as your chest and diaphragm expand, and exhale as you release all tension and stress. After several inhalations and exhalations, you will become centered and totally relaxed. Now that you're relaxed, travel with your mind and your breath to the body member that needs healing. Now inhale and exhale within the body member that you are transforming. After several times breathing in and out, a deep sense of Ma'at will emanate through the specific body part on which you are working. With each breath of renewal, you will raise your frequency and come closer and closer to reaching optimal wellness.

STEP 4—MAN HEAL THYSELF VISION QUEST

Tap into your Vision Quest and come into alignment with your higher consciousness. Be courageous; go within. Travel to uncharted territory. Stay within your breath: As you inhale, ask *the* question; and as you exhale, listen for the answer about your work, your mission. Listen for how to let go and how to embrace. Discover your purpose for being and how to arrive at your destination of greatness, of clarity, of peace. The vision may come loudly; it may even scream at you; or it may come in a whisper. Stay close, pay attention, listen, receive, then watch for the miracle as your soul releases the treasures that are within your reach.

STEP 5

Record the Findings of Your Vision Quest. Write about your meditation or vision quest in your journal. Write what guidance you received about your vision. Write the questions you still have and the plans you are making to accomplish your vision.

STEP 6

Activate "the Message"; stay on your path to your vision. Trust your inner vision; follow the guidance; move on the message. Diligently build your life's work. Embrace the treasure; manifest your prosperity. Manifest a fulfilling and prosperous life. Breathe deeper, open your eyes, and Give Thanks.

A Man Heal Thyself Man builds bridges; builds homes; builds institutes; builds his body, mind, and spirit.

BUILD YOUR VISION.
BUILD YOUR LIFE OF OPTIMAL WELLNESS.

WELLNESS WARRIOR ALTAR

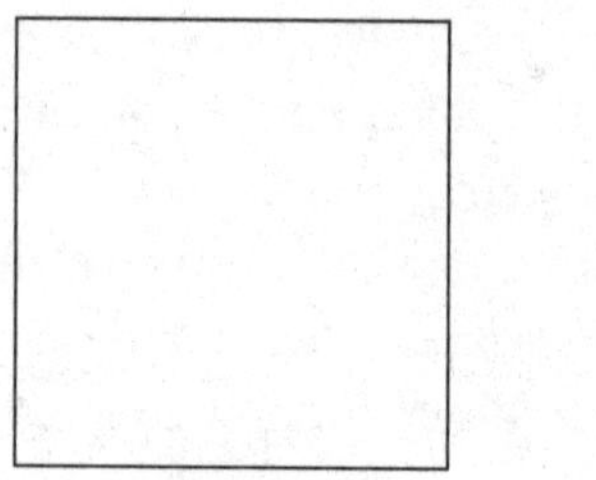

Picture of Ancestor

Picture of Most Divine Self

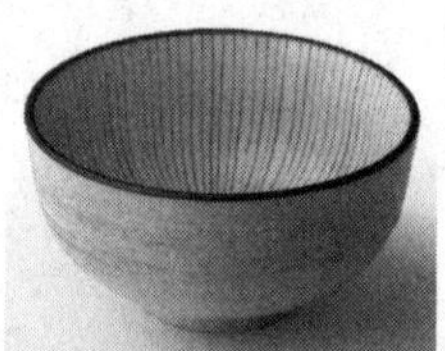

Libation Bowl

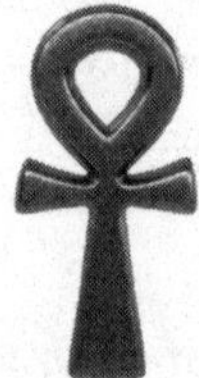

Ankh Symbol of Life and Family

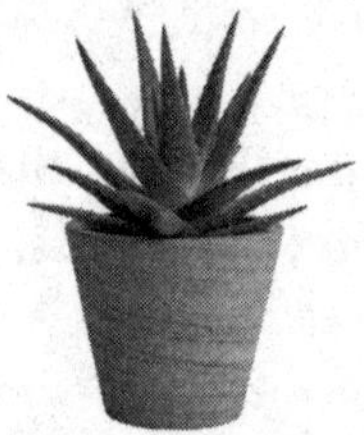

Aloe Vera Plant

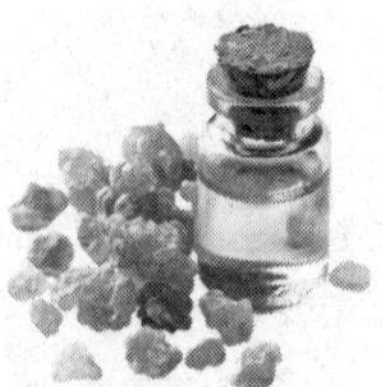

Annointing Oil: Frankincense

Candle: White or Green

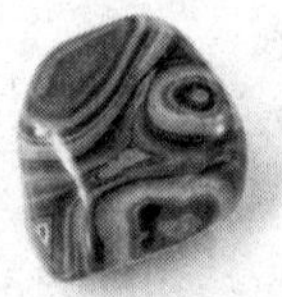

Gemstone: Malachite

Additional Optimal Altar Items for Spiritual Ascension:
White or Green Tablecloth to place over altar
Divine Instruments to be played as you pray

42 LAWS OF MA'AT

Recite the 42 Laws of Ma'at at sunrise and sunset to restore oneself to balance.

Between 4 and 6 a.m. recite:

- I will not do wrong.
- I will not steal.
- I will not act with violence.
- I will not kill.
- I will not speak unjustly.
- I will not cause pain.
- I will not waste food.
- I will not lie.
- I will not desecrate holy places.
- I will not speak evil.
- I will not abuse my sexuality.
- I will not cause the shedding of tears.
- I will not sow seeds of regret.
- I will not be an aggressor.
- I will not act guilefully.
- I will not lay waste to the ploughed land.
- I will not bear false witness.
- I will not set my mouth in motion against any person.
- I will not be wrathful and angry except for a just cause.
- I will not copulate with a man's wife.
- I will not copulate with a woman's husband.
- I will not pollute myself.
- I will not cause terror.
- I will not pollute the Earth.
- I will not speak in anger.
- I will not turn from words of right and truth.
- I will not utter curses.
- I will not initiate a quarrel.

- I will not be excitable or contentious.
- I will not prejudge.
- I will not be an eavesdropper.
- I will not speak overmuch.
- I will not commit treason against my Ancestors.
- I will not waste water.
- I will not do evil.
- I will not be arrogant.
- I will not blaspheme NTR, the One Most High (the Supreme Being).
- I will not commit fraud.
- I will not mistreat children.
- I will not mistreat animals.
- I will not defraud temple offerings.
- I will not plunder the dead.

Between 4 and 6 a.m. recite:

- I have not done wrong.
- I have not stolen.
- I have not acted with violence.
- I have not killed.
- I have not spoken unjustly.
- I have not caused pain.
- I have not wasted food.
- I have not lied.
- I have not desecrated holy places.
- I have not spoken evil.
- I have not abused my sexuality.
- I have not caused the shedding of tears.
- I have not sown seeds of regret.
- I have not been an aggressor.
- I have not acted guilefully.
- I have not lain waste to the ploughed land.
- I have not borne false witness.

- I have not set my mouth in motion against any person.
- I have not been wrathful and angry except for a just cause.
- I have not copulated with a man's wife.
- I have not copulated with a woman's husband.
- I have not polluted myself.
- I have not caused terror.
- I have not polluted the Earth.
- I have not spoken in anger.
- I have not turned from words of right and truth.
- I have not uttered curses.
- I have not initiated a quarrel.
- I have not been excitable or contentious.
- I have not prejudged.
- I have not been an eavesdropper.
- I have not spoken overmuch.
- I have not committed treason against my Ancestors.
- I have not wasted water.
- I have not done evil.
- I have not been arrogant.
- I have not blasphemed NTR, the One Most High.
- I have not committed fraud.
- I have not mistreated children.
- I have not mistreated animals.
- I have not defrauded temple offerings.
- I have not plundered the dead.

42 Laws Of Ma'at reinterpreted by Elder Master KMT Teacher Senur Ankh Ra Semahj Se Ptah

I AM A MAN—AFFIRMATIONS

I AM A MAN is dedicated to Rev. Dr. Martin Luther King Jr. and the Honorable El-Hajj Malik El-Shabazz (Malcolm X). Each was an extraordinary Optimal Man who fought, labored, marched, and spoke up for our freedom as a civil right and a human right!

OPTIMAL FREEDOM IS WELLNESS

I am free from procrastination.	I am empowered to move forward.
I am free from violence.	I am empowered to be at peace.
I am free from poverty.	I am free to acquire prosperity.
I am free from stagnation.	I am free to move forward.
I am free from destruction.	I am free to build and create greatness.
I am free from hurt and disappointment.	I am free to forgive and be forgiven.
I am free from drug addiction.	I am free to live fully and be elevated on Green Life Formula.
I am free from burdens.	I am free to release the weight of the world.
I am free from STDs.	I am empowered to live free of STDs.
I am free from premature aging.	I am empowered to reverse the aging process.
I am free from fast-food addiction.	I am empowered to embrace whole food living.
I am free from couch potato–pot belly syndrome.	I am free to be mentally and physically sound and fit.
I am free from continuing to pass on toxic DNA.	I am empowered to live disease-free.
I am free from stress.	I am empowered to embrace a calm state of serenity.

SHOUT & AFFIRM YOUR FREEDOM DAILY

ACTIVATING THE I AM PRESENCE

In the journey of self-discovery and personal growth, individuals often seek ways to connect with their inner selves and tap into their true potential. One powerful approach to this is activating the I AM presence and by daily intentional practice. By understanding and harnessing the power of the I AM presence, combined with intentional daily practices, individuals can cultivate a deeper sense of self-awareness, clarity, and purpose in their lives.

The concept of the I AM presence—originating in spiritual teachings and metaphysics—refers to the eternal, divine essence within each individual, representing their highest state of being. The I AM presence is often associated with qualities like love, wisdom, creativity, and abundance. It transcends the limitations of the ego and connects us to our true nature, allowing us to access our full potential.

Activating the I AM presence involves consciously aligning with our inner divinity and recognizing our inherent connection to the universal consciousness. Here are a few practices that can help in activating the I AM presence:

A. **MEDITATION:** Regular meditation allows us to quiet the mind, enter a state of deep relaxation, and connect with our inner self. Through meditation, we can become more attuned to the subtler aspects of our being, fostering a deeper connection with the I AM presence.

B. **AFFIRMATIONS:** Affirmations are positive statements that reinforce our desired state of being. By affirming statements such as "I am love," "I am worthy," or "I am abundant," we align our thoughts and beliefs with the qualities of the I AM presence, gradually embodying them in our daily lives.

C. **SELF-REFLECTION:** Engaging in self-reflection helps us gain insights into our thoughts, emotions, and actions. By examining our patterns and beliefs, we can identify areas that may be hindering our connection to the I AM presence. This self-awareness allows us to make conscious choices that align with our true nature.

D. **SETTING CLEAR INTENTIONS:** Begin each day by setting clear intentions for what you wish to manifest or achieve. By focusing your thoughts and energy on these intentions, you align yourself with the possibilities of the I AM presence.

E. **CULTIVATING MINDFULNESS:** Practicing mindfulness allows us to be fully present in the current moment. By paying attention to our thoughts, emotions, and surroundings without judgment, we increase our ability to make conscious choices aligned with the I AM presence.

Activating the I AM presence and being intentional daily can significantly enhance our personal growth and well-being. Intentionality is not just about thoughts; it also requires action. Take intentional steps toward your goals and aspirations, making choices that align with your core values and the qualities of the I AM presence.

By connecting with our inner divinity and aligning our thoughts, beliefs, and actions with our true nature, we tap into a wellspring of wisdom, love, and abundance. Remember that this is an ongoing practice, and consistency is key. As we integrate the power of the I AM presence and intentionality into our lives, we embark on a transformative journey toward self-realization and the fulfillment of our highest potential.

DAILY PURIFICATION POWER AFFIRMATION

Beloved Brother, this charge from Queen Afua is a gift for your 12-week rites of passage journey to Man Heal Thyself Wellness Warrior. Affirm this daily upon the rising and setting of the Sun. Be empowered! Be unified!

I have the power to create in my life what I want it
to be;
Purification of Mind, Body, and Spirit is the key!
Within this natural way of living and being,
I choose not to cut, radiate, or drug my dis-ease
away!
Instead, I cleanse, fast, juice, pray, and bless my
dis-ease away!

WHAT WE EAT

"We are what we eat."

—HONORABLE ELIJAH MOHAMMAD

"Food is not just vitamins and minerals,
food is spiritual.
Food seeks spirituality through us
and we seek spirituality through the food."

—DR. LLAILA AFRIKA

What we eat creates who we are and what we become. It refers to all the things we take into our bodies, minds, and spirits. With our bodies, we eat the food, drink the water, and breathe the air that is in our environment. Whether they are personal, social, or business-related, the relationships in our lives are ingested into our bodies, minds, and spirits. We consume our whole living experience into our whole selves, whether you are a Wounded Man or Wellness Man, your diseases or your state of wellness depends on what you consume. You are the sum total of all that you take into yourself. Figuratively and literally, "You are what you eat."

Food creates the body, builds the mind, and liberates the spirit. The higher the frequency of food ingested, the more vibrant and elevated Man becomes. As Man travels through the 12 States of Man, he will learn to consciously choose the food he will need to prevent disease and obtain optimal benefits for wellness. Eating whole organic food creates whole men free of disease.

DIETARY ENEMIES OF MAN

1. PROTEINS

UNHEALTHY FLESH:
Pork, beef, goat, lamb, chicken, and fish

RELATED DISEASES:
Numbing sensation in the extremities; cancer: prostate, colon, throat, etc.; kidney failure; enlarged testicles; and toxic sperm

DIETARY WELLNESS PROTEIN ALTERNATIVES:
TVP (textured vegetable protein), beans, lentils, sprouts, raw nuts, seeds, and Queen Afua Green Life Nutritional Formula

2. CARBOHYDRATES

UNHEALTHY CARBS:
White rice, white bread, and white potatoes

RELATED DISEASES:
Constipation, abdominal bloating, gas, and shortness of breath

DIETARY WELLNESS CARB ALTERNATIVES:
Sprouted bread, brown rice, couscous, bulgur wheat, tabouli, and buckwheat pancakes

3. FATS/OILS

UNHEALTHY FATS/OILS:
Polyunsaturated fats, trans-fats, and saturated fats

RELATED DISEASES:
High blood pressure, stroke, numbness sensation, and sluggishness

DIETARY WELLNESS FATS/OILS ALTERNATIVES:
Cold-pressed olive oil, sesame oil, and cold-pressed flaxseed oil

4. CALCIUM

UNHEALTHY DAIRY:
Milk, cheese, ice cream, butter, eggs, and yogurt

RELATED DISEASES:
Constipation, clogged arteries, respiratory issues, blockages, asthma, colds, allergies, snoring, and toxic/acidic sperm

DIETARY WELLNESS DAIRY ALTERNATIVES:
Almond milk, sesame milk, and green vegetable juice

5. SWEETS

UNHEALTHY SUGAR:
Corn syrup, fructose, brown and white sugar

RELATED DISEASES:
Diabetes, stress, arthritis aches and pains, headaches, depression, mood swings, and devitalized weak sperm

DIETARY WELLNESS SWEET ALTERNATIVES:
Licorice root, raw honey, dates, raisins, currants, agave, and stevia

6. SALT

UNHEALTHY SALT:
Iodized salt

RELATED DISEASES:
High blood pressure, stroke, and impotence

DIETARY WELLNESS SALT ALTERNATIVES:
Sea salt, kelp, dulse, and nori

7. INGESTIBLE ENEMIES OF MAN:
Drugs, alcohol, cigarettes, soft drinks, and coffee

RELATED DISEASES:
Shortened life span, weakened immune system, damaged liver and lungs, devitalized weak sperm

WELLNESS ALTERNATIVES TO USING INGESTIBLE ENEMIES:
Invert body for 10 minutes, write in your Journal, recite Man Heal Thyself Daily Declarations and Affirmations, rise between 4 a.m. and 5 a.m. and Perform Manifestation Practice to integrate the wellness regime with the elements of your wellness (Air, Fire, Water, Earth) (see chapter 2)

8. OTHER DIETARY ENEMIES

(THE PATHWAY TO AN IMPOTENT LIFE):
Genetically engineered foods; microwaved foods; fried foods; pasteurized foods; chemically saturated fruits, nuts, grains, and beans

RELATED DISEASES:
Chronic fatigue, numbing, mean-spiritedness, hostility, depression, devitalized weak sperm

WELLNESS ALTERNATIVES TO OTHER DIETARY ENEMIES:
Incorporate holistic tools and strategies into your daily lifestyle. Follow the instructions provided on the Man Heal Thyself Scrolls (Charts)

SETTING UP YOUR NUTRITION KITCHEN HEALING LABORATORY

As you begin your detox plan, you should prepare your environment. Below are some things you may need to obtain to set up your kitchen as a laboratory for creating your wellness.

ITEMS YOU WILL NEED TO FACILITATE CONVERTING YOUR KITCHEN INTO A HEALING LABORATORY:

JUICER: to juice live fruits and vegetables
BLENDER: to blend juices, sauces, and nutrients
STAINLESS STEEL POTS: for preparing steamed vegetables and herbal teas
CHARTS AND PRODUCTS: See websites for Queen Afua and Heal Thyself charts and products positioned throughout this text

Also consider:

FOOD PROCESSOR: for preparing vegetables to make soups and salads

DEHYDRATOR: for preparing live cookies, croquettes, pie fillings, veggie chips

SPROUTER: for growing your own alfalfa sprouts, mung bean sprouts, broccoli sprouts

NOTE: As stated at the opening of this book, if you are presently consulting a physician for existing health challenges, CONTINUE to follow the advice of your physician. The information provided here is designed to be inspirational and help you make informed decisions about your health. This material is NOT intended to be a substitute for any medical advice or treatment that has been prescribed by your physician.

Use the tools in your kitchen laboratory and your charts (The City of Wellness Nutrition Kitchen and Pyramids of Wellness) to plan your meals. Consult your Man Heal Thyself Scroll to plan the rest of your holistic Wellness Life.

These are basic steps or levels of food consumption. Most people's food plan exists on more than one of them. To detox and rejuvenate, try to prepare, eat, and drink one step higher than your present level. For optimal wellness, follow the Advanced Juice Fast for 7 consecutive days as you travel on your 12-week journey.

WEEKS 1–3

LEVEL 1—BEGINNER—FLEXITARIAN

The Family Man | The Sensual Man | The Transformation Man

Consume vegetable protein as well as organic chicken and unshelled fish. Incorporate beans, peas, sprouts, and lentils into your diet. Omit all other flesh foods (beef, pork, lamb, turkey, goat, etc.). Consume more fresh fruit, vegetables, and whole grains.

WEEKS 4–6

LEVEL 2—INTERMEDIATE—VEGETARIAN

The Lover Man | The Communication Man | The Intuitive Man

Consume only vegetarian foods. Omit all flesh foods (seafood, beef, pork, lamb, turkey, goat, etc.). Fresh vegetable intake should include 50 percent or 75 percent live food and 50 percent or 25 percent steamed food to retain as much of the live enzymes and oxygen as possible.

WEEKS 7–9

LEVEL 3—ADVANCED VEGAN (RAW)

The Universal Man | The Illuminated Man | The Harmonizing Man

Consume 100 percent live, uncooked food. Live food includes organic live proteins (sprouted beans, raw soaked nuts and seeds, avocados), live soups, uncooked grains such as couscous, tabouli, bulgur wheat, etc. Consume whole or juiced fresh fruits and vegetables. Drink daily 8 ounces of warm water, 5 cups Herbal Master Tea, and 8 ounces of Kidney-Liver Flush.

WEEKS 10–12

LEVEL 4—ADVANCED
WHOLE FOOD THERAPEUTIC JUICE FAST

The Nature Man | The Alchemist Man | The Supreme Man

Consume 100 percent organic liquid meals only. This cleansing-level meal consists daily of 2 vegetable juice meals for rejuvenation and 1 fruit meal for detoxification. Additionally, there is a daily intake of ½ gallon warm water, 5 cups Herbal Master Tea, and 8 ounces of Kidney-Liver Flush. LEVEL 4 is a therapeutic juice fast that should be followed for 7 days each season (84 days). Elements of the juice fast are part of all four steps.

MAN HEAL THYSELF 12-WEEK WORKOUT PLAN

INSTRUCTIONS

The 12-week workout plan incorporates a set of 9 exercises for Monday through Friday. At home, no gym. Each week, add 5 reps to each exercise for 12 weeks.

See a breakdown of exercises below.

MONDAY

- 20 squats
- 15-second plank
- 25 crunches
- 35 jumping jacks
- 15 lunges
- 25-second wall sit
- 10 sit-ups
- 10 butt kicks
- 5 push-ups

TUESDAY

- 10 squats
- 30-second plank
- 25 crunches
- 10 jumping jacks
- 25 lunges
- 45-second wall sit
- 35 sit-ups
- 25 butt kicks
- 10 push-ups

WEDNESDAY
- 15 squats
- 40-second plank
- 30 crunches
- 50 jumping jacks
- 25 lunges
- 35-second wall sit
- 30 sit-ups
- 25 butt kicks
- 10 push-ups

THURSDAY
- 35 squats
- 30-second plank
- 20 crunches
- 25 jumping jacks
- 15 lunges
- 60-second wall sit
- 55 sit-ups
- 33 butt kicks
- 20 push-ups

FRIDAY
- 25 squats
- 60-second plank
- 30 crunches
- 55 jumping jacks
- 60 lunges
- 45-second wall sit
- 40 sit-ups
- 50 butt kicks
- 30 push-ups

Repeat these circuits 2 or 3 times, with 1 minute rest between series.

Saturday and Sunday are rest days.

CARDIO

1ST WEEK: 5 sets of a 30-second sprint followed by a 30-second jog

2ND WEEK: 6 sets of a 35-second sprint followed by a 45-second jog

3RD WEEK: 7 sets of a 45-second sprint followed by a 60-second jog

4TH WEEK: 8 sets of a 50-second sprint followed by a 45-second jog

5TH WEEK: 7 sets of a 55-second sprint followed by a 30-second jog

6TH WEEK: 6 sets of a 60-second sprint followed by a 45-second jog

7TH WEEK: 5 sets of a 65-second sprint followed by a 60-second jog

8TH WEEK: 6 sets of a 70-second sprint followed by a 45-second jog

9TH WEEK: 7 sets of a 75-second sprint followed by a 30-second jog

10TH WEEK: 8 sets of an 80-second sprint followed by a 45-second jog

11TH WEEK: 7 sets of an 85-second sprint followed by a 50-second jog

12TH WEEK: 8 sets of a 90-second sprint followed by a 55-second jog

WEEKLY CHECK-UP CHART

(SAMPLE)

Check off your progress on your path to Optimal Wellness.

SUNRISE WELLNESS

	Day 1	Day 2	Day 3	Day 4	Day 5	Day 6	Day 7
Recite/Reflect on Affirmations from Antiquity							
Drink the juice of lemons and 16 oz warm water with 2 tbsp colon base							
Invert body for 10 minutes							

Green Life Liquid Breakfast (8 oz fresh juice with 8 oz water + 1–2 tbsp of Green Life)							
Liquid Meal 30 minutes later							
Solid Meal, Drink Master Herbal Formula							
Complete Daily Workout							

MIDDAY WELLNESS (Lunch)

	Day 1	Day 2	Day 3	Day 4	Day 5	Day 6	Day 7
Green Life Liquid Lunch (8–16 oz fresh juice or water with 1–2 tbsp of Green Life)							
Solid Vegan Lunch: Green Power Lunch (salad/ steamed vegetables/ whole grains/protein, e.g., beans, lentils)							

Flexitarian Lunch: Steamed fish as protein with vegetables and whole grains							

SUNSET WELLNESS (Dinner)

	Day 1	Day 2	Day 3	Day 4	Day 5	Day 6	Day 7
Liquid Dinner, Green Life Nutritional Dinner (8–16 oz vegetable juice and water with 1–2 tbsp Green Life Nutritional Formula)							
Green Power Dinner (salad/steamed vegetables/whole grains/protein, e.g., beans, peas, lentils)							
Flexitarian Dinner: Steamed fish as protein with vegetables and whole grains							

Man Life Herbal Tonic (7 days) alternate with Master Herbal Tonic (7 days). Directions: Add 6 tbsp to 4 oz boiling water and let steep for 1 hr (off the stove). Drink before bedtime.							
Take 3 Herbal Laxative Tablets							
Detox Bath: Fill a tub with warm water and add 1 to 2 lbs Epsom salt. Soak for 30 minutes.							
Zone Body Massage: body, face, hands							
Apply clay over the body member in need overnight							

MAN HEAL THYSELF JOURNAL PAGE

(SAMPLE)

Prepare to record your journey to wellness.

Purchase or prepare a notebook to record your experiences of transformation to wellness of body, mind, and spirit.

VISION QUEST JOURNAL PAGE

RISE | SHINE | LISTEN | RECEIVE | ACTIVATE

____

____

____

____

____

____

____

____

____

____

____

THE POWER TO HEAL IS WITHIN

BUILDING LEAN BODY MASS WITH PLANT-BASED NUTRITION

Individuals seeking healthier and more sustainable dietary alternatives are developing a growing interest in plant-based nutrition, inspired by the significant number of celebrities and influencers and as evidenced by the growth of the health and wellness industries (currently generating hundreds of billions of dollars annually). Contrary to the misconception that plant-based diets may hinder muscle growth, emerging research indicates that it is indeed possible to build lean body mass while following a plant-based lifestyle.

A common concern with plant-based diets is whether they provide sufficient protein for muscle building. However, research suggests that most individuals, including athletes, can meet their needs for this vital element through plant-based sources. The American Dietetic Association states that well-planned vegetarian and vegan diets can provide adequate protein for all stages of life, including periods of intense physical activity.

Legumes such as lentils, chickpeas, and black beans are rich in protein, fiber, and essential amino acids necessary for muscle repair and growth. Additionally, sprouted tofu, tempeh, and seitan serve as excellent plant-based protein alternatives in moderation. These sources of rich antioxidants and phytonutrients are often low in saturated fat, aiding in maintaining a healthy body composition and improved cardiovascular health. By combining a variety of these foods throughout the day, individuals can ensure they receive the essential amino acids necessary for muscle synthesis.

Numerous athletes have successfully adopted plant-based diets while building and sustaining lean body mass. The success of athletes like tennis champion Novak Djokovic, ultra-endurance athlete Scott Jurek, and Olympic weightlifter Kendrick Farris exemplifies the potential of plant-based nutrition for athletic performance and muscle development. Their achievements debunk the myth that animal-based protein is necessary for optimal muscle growth.

Here are 20 tips for building lean muscle mass through plant-based vegan and strength-training protocols:

1. Focus on consuming a variety of plant-based protein sources such as legumes, tempeh, seitan, quinoa, and hemp seeds throughout your day.
2. Make sure to eat enough calories to support muscle growth by including energy-dense foods like nuts, seeds, avocados, and whole grains in your diet.
3. Prioritize whole, minimally processed foods to ensure you're getting a wide range of nutrients.
4. Consume adequate amounts of carbohydrates to fuel your workouts and aid in muscle recovery. Good sources include fruits: bananas, raisins; vegetables: red potatoes, yams; and whole grains: quinoa, sprouted brown rice, wild rice.
5. Include healthy fats in your diet, such as avocados, nuts, and olive oil, as they support hormone production and provide energy.
6. Stay hydrated by drinking plenty of water throughout the day, as it aids in muscle function and recovery.
7. Incorporate strength-training exercises into your routine to stimulate muscle growth. Focus on compound exercises like squats, deadlifts, bench presses, and rows.
8. To continually challenge your muscles, gradually increase the intensity and weight of your workouts as your strength improves.
9. Consider incorporating resistance bands or bodyweight exercises into your routine for added variety and muscle engagement.
10. Prioritize proper form and technique during your workouts to maximize muscle activation and minimize the risk of injury.
11. Incorporate high-intensity interval training (HIIT) into your rou-

tine to increase cardiovascular fitness and promote fat loss while maintaining muscle mass.

12. Engage in regular stretching and mobility exercises to improve flexibility and prevent muscle imbalances.
13. Allow for adequate rest and recovery between workouts to give your muscles time to repair and grow.
14. Consume a post-workout meal or snack containing a combination of protein and carbohydrates to aid in muscle recovery and glycogen replenishment.
15. Include foods rich in vitamins and minerals, such as leafy greens, berries, and citrus fruits, to support overall health and muscle function.
16. Experiment with different plant-based protein powders or supplements, such as pea protein, hemp, or sprouted brown rice protein, to supplement your protein intake if needed.
17. Aim for at least 7 to 8 hours of quality sleep each night, as sleep plays a crucial role in muscle recovery and growth.
18. Consider working with a qualified vegan nutritionist or dietitian to ensure you're meeting your nutritional needs for muscle growth.
19. Stay consistent with your training and nutrition plan, as building lean muscle mass takes time and dedication.
20. Listen to your body and adjust your training and nutrition based on how you feel and the progress you're making.

This Workbook section provides instructions for using tools and strategies for wellness that are suggested throughout the book. Remember, it's always a good idea to consult with a health-care professional or certified trainer before starting any new exercise or diet program.

CHAPTER 5

MAN OF VITALITY

ARIT STATE 1:
THE FAMILY MAN OF UNITY AND WEALTH

ARIT STATE 2:
THE SENSUAL MAN OF HEIGHTENED SENSITIVITY

ARIT STATE 3:
THE TRANSFORMATION MAN OF RENEWAL

ARIT STATE 4:
THE LOVER MAN OF HARMONY

ARIT STATE 5:
THE COMMUNICATION MAN OF CONNECTIVITY AND CREATIVITY

ARIT STATE 6:
THE INTUITIVE MAN OF CLEAR VISION

ARIT STATE 7:
THE UNIVERSAL HUMANITARIAN MAN

"Arrange for me the way.
May I renew myself.
May I become strong."

—THE PAPYRUS OF ANI

WHAT ARE THE ARITU?

The Aritu and the chakras are one and the same. Aritu is the original name that was born out of Afri-Khametic teachings. The word *chakra*, as an extension of that, was born out of Hindu teachings.

The Arit or Aritu (plural) are energy centers within the human body. They are the same as the chakra system (from the East Indian spiritual tradition), which can be represented as wheels of flowers or wheels of light. They are round and approximately 1 foot in diameter. When the body is vibrant and healthy, the Aritu spin clockwise. When the body is toxic, the Aritu spin counterclockwise. An Arit is a spiritual center that communicates by sending messages and signals to the body. It is encoded with information about the lifetimes of one's being, essentially functioning like a reference library or a time capsule. The information can reach the physical and mental bodies according to the condition of the Arit. The Aritu also function like a lighthouse that radiates frequencies and electrical currents that register as high or low, determining the frequency of the body, mind, and spirit. If the Arit's energy is high, one will enjoy optimal wellness. If the Arit's energy is low, the individual will suffer from poor health. The Arit contains within itself the masculine hemisphere of consciousness, which rules material, intellectual, and financial conditions. The feminine consciousness rules the spiritual, creative, and intuitive side of man. As one journeys through the 12 Aritu, or states of man, and applies Man Heal Thyself practices of meditation, affirmation, food as medicine, self-massage, breathing exercises, herbology, and elemental healing (healing with earth, air, fire, and water), man will bring himself into an optimal state of well-being.

MAN HEAL THYSELF WELLNESS WARRIOR SCROLLS

The Man Heal Thyself Wellness Warrior Scrolls are located within the first 7 Aritu of this text. These Scrolls are road maps that holistically and actively guide yourself to Wellness. Apply the work of the Scrolls to restore your body with strategies for using food as medicine, as well as affirmations, power charges, meditations, and body work. The Scrolls are intended to be additional tools to reach your goal of purifying and restoring all the parts of yourself. When you work to bring dynamic wellness and harmony to your whole anatomy—body, mind, and spirit—you can become like a concert of the richest sound. Wellness Warrior Salute!

DEFINITIONS OF CATEGORIES USED ON THE MAN HEAL THYSELF WELLNESS WARRIOR SCROLLS:

Man Heal Thyself Wellness Warrior deals with the total male anatomy. Focus on the anatomy connected to the specific Arit you are working with to detoxify and to rejuvenate for 7 to 12 weeks.

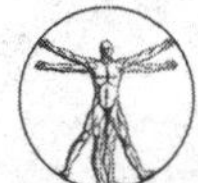

Support this divine calling with the Man Heal Thyself Wellness Warrior lifestyle and you will restore thyself. Remember every day that the power to heal is within.

ANTIQUITY AFFIRMATION:

Perform a daily meditation at sunrise and sunset. Sit quietly and recite the Antiquity Affirmation or an affirmation of choice. As you speak, you become what you speak. Speak yourself into existence. Recite affirmations to awaken your "dry bones." Resurrect yourself with each word. The Antiquity Affirmations are all based on the Nile Valley of KMT Healing Affirmations from the first civilization. Light a white candle and light up your heart. Allow the ancient ones, the shining beings, to shine through as you speak your body temple into wakefulness.

METAPHYSICAL WELLNESS CHARGE:

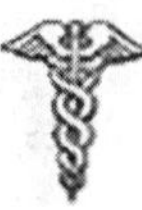

Thoughts are things that we think in our mental body (mind) and feel as well as create in our physical bodies. We can reshape our lives by the transformation of our minds. This section features a power charge to be spoken daily. Each day, use your words to bring forth what you need to bring your body temple to wholeness and healing.

SPIRITUAL AND PHYSICAL DISEASES:

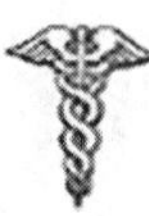

Disease manifests spiritually before it takes root physically. Each part of our anatomy is imbued with divinity. This section details the corresponding physical area(s) for the respective Arit (chakra). Use this section to further educate yourself and know yourself.

HERBAL COMPOUND:

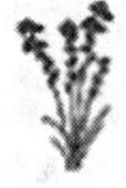

If you have a chronic disease, for 1 to 3 weeks take the specific herbal compound that supports recovery of the specific body member. Boil 3 cups of water at night, turn off the flame, and then add 3 teaspoons of each loose herb. Cover the pot and steep overnight.

In the morning, strain the tea, then drink before noon.

Loose Herbs:

—Steep 1 teaspoon of loose herbs in 1 cup of distilled water. Strain and drink.

Powdered Herbs:

—Steep ¼ teaspoon of herbal powder in 1 cup of distilled water. Strain and drink.

Tinctures:

Add 10 drops of your tincture to 1 cup of distilled water. Strain and drink. Nurture yourself with nature by drinking your tonics. Bathe yourself in bath water you fortify either with Epsom salts or a tonic you make by mixing 2 tablespoons of Queen Afua Master Herbal Formula into apple cider vinegar. Then massage yourself with olive oil, castor oil, or almond oil to bring harmony to the psychological, emotional, and physical parts of your anatomy.

NATURE'S CURE:

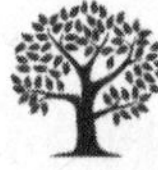

"Food as medicine" recipes to be eaten daily throughout that respective week.

CLAY POULTICE:

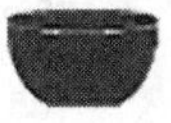

For 3 to 7 weeks, apply a 1-inch poultice (clay pack) over the areas of the body that are swollen, inflamed, or in pain. Cover the ends of the gauze with nonsurgical tape to keep gauze in place.

Leave the poultice on overnight. In the morning, take a warm shower.

ZONE MASSAGE:

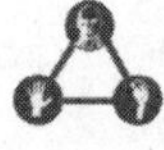

There are reflexology points on the face, hands, and feet that connect to the organs and systems (respiratory, circulatory, etc.) of the body. Massaging of the reflexology points stimulates blood flow to the related body part and/or system.

Anatomy of Man	Antiquity Affirmation	Wellness Power Charge	Spiritual & Physical Diseases
"I am a shining being. I have been created by and have come into existence from the Most High."	*"I speak that I wish to become strong and it comes into being as I speak."*	*"Arrange for me the way. May I renew myself. May I become strong."*	*"I am glorious, I am pure."*
Skin Meditate and breathe deeply as you fill your skin with the light of purity.	"May I see my beauty. May I advance upon the Earth. Tehuti (Divine Inner Intelligence) protects my flesh entirely."	"I release all penned-up emotions that cause disease!"	**Spiritual Disease** Rage, resentment, anger **Physical Disease** Eczema, blackheads, shingles, boils
Legs and Feet Meditate and breathe deeply as you fill your legs and feet with the light of the full moon.	"Make strong my legs to rise up for me. I have gained power over my feet. May I stretch my feet which are fastened together."	"I am free to move to higher ground!"	**Spiritual Disease** Inability to move forward or to learn from lessons **Physical Disease** Water retention, swollen legs, feet, and ankles

Muscular System Meditate and breathe deeply as you fill your muscular system with the light of strength.	"I shall not be seized by my arms, nor shall I be carried away by my hands, nor shall I allow anyone to bring harm to me."	"I am strengthened through every challenge!"	**Spiritual Disease** Lack of self-control **Physical Disease** Sore, aching muscles
Bones Meditate and breathe deeply as you fill your bones with hope.	"I come into being from unformed matter. Make me always prosperous. Triumphantly gather my bones and collect my limbs."	"I move in strength!"	**Spiritual Disease** Fearful of the unknown, shattered dreams, broken vision **Physical Disease** Arthritis, tooth decay, swollen joints

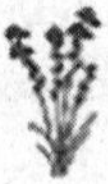 Herbal Compound	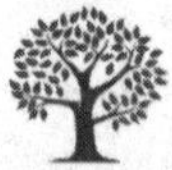 Nature Cure	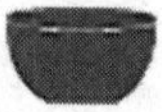 Clay Cure	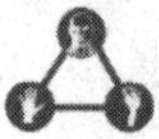 Zone Massage
"I come into being from unformed matter. I grow into the form of plants."	*"An ounce of prevention is worth a pound of cure."*	*"In the beginning, the Most High gave every people a cup of clay and they drank their life." From Proverbs of Digger Indians*	*"I am the knot within the olive tree."*
Aloe, burdock, sarsaparilla: Drink as an herbal tea and use as an herbal bath.	Mix equal parts of organic oatmeal and cornmeal with water, and scrub skin with loofah brush. Then wash and shower.	Apply Heal Thyself Rejuvenation Clay over skin and let air-dry for 1 hour. Take a bath and add 1–2 lbs of salt (or apple cider vinegar if you have high blood pressure).	**Face:** Massage the jawbone on both sides of the face. **Hands:** Massage the padding of each hand. **Feet:** Massage the heels of each foot.

Ginger, cornsilk, bladderwrack	Eat and drink from the berry family (cranberries, raspberries, blueberries, etc.). Add 1 teabag of Goldenseal or Aloe to a tub of warm water and take a 30-minute bath.	Apply Heal Thyself Rejuvenation Clay to gauze, place over legs and feet where there is pain, and leave on overnight. Take a warm shower in the morning. Complete this process 3 times a week.	**Face:** Massage the jawbone on each side of the face. **Hands:** Massage the padding of each hand. **Feet:** Massage the heels of each foot.
Arnica cream, wintergreen oil, or birch oil for massaging	Increase vegetable protein (beans, lentils, soaked nuts, etc.). Add 1 tbsp of Green Life Nutritional Formula to 8–12 oz distilled water and drink 3 times a day.	Apply Heal Thyself Rejuvenation Clay to gauze, place over legs and feet where there is pain, and leave on overnight. Take a warm shower in the morning. Complete this process 3 times a week.	**Face:** Full face massage. **Hands:** Full hand massage. **Feet:** Full foot massage.

Herbal Compound	Nature Cure	Clay Cure	Zone Massage
Boneset, horsetail, yucca, alfalfa	Juice ½ cup of fresh turnips with 8 oz of dark vegetable juice.	Apply Heal Thyself Rejuvenation Clay to gauze, place over painful bones and joints, and leave on overnight. Take a shower in the morning and wash your body. Complete this process at least 3 times a week	**Face:** Massage jawbone for general stimulation. **Hands:** Massage fingers on both hands for general stimulation. **Feet:** Massage toes on both feet for general stimulation.

DAILY SPIRITUAL OBSERVANCES

The following Spiritual Observances are to be practiced by each man from the beginning of his Man Heal Thyself Wellness Warrior journey. See each separate ARIT section for additional SPIRITUAL OBSERVANCES assignments.

ARIT POWER CENTER: (1–12)

ARIT COLOR: (1–12)

ITEMS YOU WILL NEED TO FACILITATE SPIRITUAL OBSERVANCES:

EPSOM OR DEAD SEA SALTS: for spiritual baths to recall the ocean

SACRED INSTRUMENT: bell, drum, sitar, shekere, etc., to awaken the in-dwelling agent host

PURIFIED OR ALKALINE WATER: to offer libation

JOURNAL: to record spiritual messages received

PREVIOUSLY MADE TONICS: See page 20

PREVIOUSLY GATHERED ALTAR MATERIALS: See page 34

- **THERAPEUTIC-GRADE ESSENTIAL OILS**
- **CUP OR BOWL FOR LIBATION**
- **CANDLES, INCENSE**
- **HEALING STONE (MALACHITE)**

1. THE SPIRITUAL BATH

- Begin your journey into the Arit by entering the depths of the ocean. One way to honor this intention is to create a dawn ritual of taking a spiritual bath with Epsom salts or Dead Sea salts when you rise between the hours of 4 a.m. and 6 a.m.
- Make a ceremony out of your bath. Light candles and incense; have soft, inspiring music playing. Bless your bathwater. Use the bath to release all negativity,

everything that blocks the free movement of light, love, healing, and peace through your Body Temple.

- Place 7 drops of the essential oils of frankincense and myrrh into the bathwater to open your crown Arit (chakra). Frankincense and myrrh attune you to the Divine Oneness of NTR inspiration and divine wisdom. They bring forth the Divinity and holistic and metaphysical empowerment. Frankincense and myrrh help to eliminate confusion and depression by easing anxiety and stress. Also, each contains antiseptic, antibacterial, and anti-inflammatory properties.
- Select only pure therapeutic-grade essential oils.

2. AROMATHERAPY

- Add several drops of frankincense and myrrh oil to a diffuser each morning to purify yourself and your sacred prayer space. Select only pure therapeutic-grade essential oils.

3. YOUR ALTAR

- Set up your altar according to the Man Heal Thyself Wellness Warrior altar preparation guidelines (see page 34). Sit before your altar quietly and meditatively on the floor or in a comfortable chair. Add 7 drops of frankincense and myrrh oil to a bowl of purified or alkaline water on your altar and sprinkle a few drops around your prayer space.
- **Anoint with Frankincense and Myrrh Oils:** Select only therapeutic-grade essential oils. Use essential oils of frankincense and myrrh to anoint your **CROWN** and your **THIRD EYE** (in the center of your forehead between your eyebrows), the Body Temple doorway of supreme spirituality. Next, anoint your **HEART**, the Body Temple doorway of compassion and divine love.

Also anoint your **PROSTATE AREA**, the **PALMS OF YOUR HANDS** to make everything you touch more sacred, and the **BOTTOMS OF YOUR FEET** to spiritually align yourself for stepping out in power, promise, and faith.

- **Sacred Musical Instrument:** Softly play a sacred instrument (drum, sistrum, shekere) to awaken the in-dwelling angelic host. Or you might want to use a small, clear-toned bell at that early hour out of respect for the others sleeping in your household.

4. AFFIRMATION FOR ARIT

See Arit appropriate to the week you are in.

5. LIBATION:

A libation is the act of pouring a liquid such as water or spirits (alcohol) as a holy offering to the One Creator. In Man Heal Thyself Wellness Warrior practices, we use purified or alkaline water that we have blessed and offered ceremonially to the Most High.

First, take a sip of water in honor of yourself and the inner work you are accomplishing to achieve unity, harmony, and abundance within yourself as well as for your family. Take another sip for holistic and metaphysical empowerment of your Arit Power Center.

For the libation, pour a small amount of water from a cup, bowl, or calabash bowl, or sprinkle a few drops with your fingers onto a potted plant on your altar or onto the earth if you are outside. As you pour your libation, call out this Prayer of Adoration: *I pour this libation in praise and adoration of the Most High, the One Creator* (or name you use). *I pour this libation in praise and adoration of myself,* (state your name). *I pour this libation in praise and adoration of my ancestors,* (state their names).

6. **MAN HEAL THYSELF WELLNESS WARRIOR PRAYER:**

May I open my two eyes which are blind
May I stretch out my feet which are fastened together
May my legs be strong and raise me up
I know my heart
I have gained power over my hands and arms
I have gained power over my two feet
I have gained the power to do what pleaseth my soul
May my body and soul not be imprisoned
I rise and shine . . .
I am powerful. I am mighty.
I come forth in peace.

—THE PAPYRUS OF ANI

7. **EMPOWERMENT AND DETOXIFICATION AFFIRMATION**

See Arit appropriate to the week you are in.

8. **CHANT (HESI):**

Chant this hesi 7 times daily for external exultation and proclamation.
MAKERU—Victory
Chant this hesi 7 times daily for internal invocation and exultation.
NUK PU MAKERU—I Am Victorious

9. **FIRE BREATHS:**

Prepare for your Fire Breathing (rapid breathing) by slowly inhaling 4 times and slowly exhaling 4 times.
When you are totally at ease, begin your fire breaths.
Allow each deep Fire Breath to represent the opening of your crown Arit (chakra) to connect to the Most High through illumination and empowerment.
In Arit 11, you will complete 1,100 Fire Breaths.
With each new Arit, you will add 100 more Fire Breaths.

By Arit 12, you will be performing 1,200 breaths of power and light.

How to Do Fire Breaths:

- Drink a glass of purified or alkaline water.
- Place a few drops of Queen Afua Breath of Life (organic eucalyptus and organic peppermint oils) under your tongue.
- Sit up straight and tall, lengthening the space between your belly button and heart.
- With your mouth closed, breath in and out through your nose, pulling your abdomen in during the exhale and pressing your abdomen out during your inhale.
- Inhale deeply like a pump, imagining your belly filling up with air during the inhale and using your abdominal muscles to push the air out during the exhale.
- Practice the Fire Breath a few times slowly.
- Start to shorten each breath and pick up the pace. Fire Breaths should be loud and quick.
- Equalize your inhale and exhale in both strength and length.
- Make sure, after you complete your Fire Breaths, to pause and take a few smooth, deep breaths as you enjoy the benefits of Fire Breathing.

Please Note:

- If you should become light-headed or slightly breathless, which is called hyperventilating, simply breathe into a small paper bag—**NOT** plastic—held over your nose and mouth for a few minutes to restore your carbon dioxide balance.
- Your nose might start to run from the release of congestion from Fire Breathing. So you might want to have a few tissues nearby in case.

10. HEALING STONE MEDITATION AND VISUALIZATION

HEALING STONE = MALACHITE

Malachite is a green stone of protection that is often referred to as a stone of transformation and personal growth, encouraging the release of past traumas, old emotional patterns, and suppressed feelings in order to step out of one's comfort zone. Malachite clears and activates the Aritu (chakras) while attuning to spiritual guidance. Malachite aids in balancing and calming all those who encounter it. This stone energizes the fourth Arit (chakra), which regulates the heart center, seat of love and compassion.

How to visualize

- Place malachite stone by your heart for spiritual restoration. Inhale deep into your heart, then make a deep exhalation from the heart. The heart is reflected in Ma'atian African Consciousness, which represents balance, truth, and wholeness.
- Take 4 deep, heart-healing breaths. See your heart, your relationships, your inner harmony awaken from within. Then relax your palms, placing them upward with your stone in hand, and visualize your body, mind, and spirit becoming as light as a feather. Be without anger or judgment—only peace and serenity will permeate your entire Body Temple.
- Increase the length of time you spend in meditation every 7 days. The longer you are in meditation, the deeper your inner peace will be. The more solid your ba (spirit) will become. The cleaner your Body Temple, the sooner it will be able to live permanently in the peace and inner balance of the meditative state.

11. HERBAL TONICS:

- Drink daily Queen Afua Master Herbal Formula to detoxify your entire Body Temple.

  —OR—
- Drink daily Man Heal Thyself Man's Life Herbal Formula to rejuvenate and detoxify the prostate.

  —OR—
- Drink daily the herbal compound of the week to support specific organ groups (see Herbs on Scrolls, page 62).
- Boil 3 cups of water between 8 p.m. and 9 p.m. in the evening. Add 2 to 3 teaspoons per herb, and let steep overnight for a potent herbal blend. By the morning, strain and drink by 12 p.m. Refrigerate and don't reheat.

12. WELLNESS WARRIOR JOURNAL WRITING

Journal writing is best done after your spiritual bath and/or internal cleansing (with an enema), and/or meditation. When you are cleansed and centered, you can receive spiritual messages from the One Most High with empowerment. When in the spirit, messages travel down through your spirit mind, to your heart, into your hand, and onto the paper.

The best time to receive your spiritually written work is after you have completed your altar work, between the hours of 4 a.m. and 6 a.m. Keep a special pen and journal by or on your altar to work with the power, force, and stillness at the coming of dawn.

Affirm your daily life. At this time, write in your journal thoughts, activities, experiences, and interactions that present themselves. You can also write down your visions, desires, dreams, and affirmations so that you will be able to draw on these resources when help and support are most needed.

13. **AFFIRMATION CONFIRMATION:**

At the beginning of Arit 1, you created a personal Affirmation Confirmation.

- Take a few moments to affirm yourself daily.
- Affirm yourself in the morning when you rise and in the night before you fall into slumber.
- Both in the morning and in the night, repeat your Affirmation Confirmation to yourself 3 times: 1 time for your mind, 1 time for your body, and 1 time for your spirit.

14. **PRAYER OF FORGIVENESS:**

At the beginning of Arit 1, you created a personal Prayer of Forgiveness.

- Take a few moments to say your Prayer of Forgiveness daily.
- Pray at least once a day.

15. **PROBLEM-SOLVER AFFIRMATIONS:**

Affirm and repeat 3 times each:

I am a problem-solver!

I solve problems!

I am the master of solving problems! I am a master of life's mathematics! I do not run from problems because I am the problem-solver!

Whatever is thrown at me, I can solve.

16. **VALUE AND POWER AFFIRMATIONS:**

Affirm and repeat three times each:

I will not negotiate my value and power!

I stand affirmed and absolute!
I affirm love, potential, and healing!
I will not negotiate my light!
I will not dumb down my value!
I am open to receive my divine complement that reflects my sacred value of self! I will charge into my life what it will be.

17. CHARGE AFFIRMATION CONFIRMATION:

At the beginning of Arit 3, you created a personal Accountability Power Charge Affirmation Confirmation.

- Take a few moments to affirm yourself daily.
- Affirm yourself in the morning when you rise and in the night before you fall into slumber.
- Both in the morning and in the night, repeat your Accountability Power Charge Affirmation Confirmation to yourself 3 times: 1 time for your mind, 1 time for your body, and 1 time for your spirit.

18. LOVE AFFIRMATIONS:

Affirm and repeat 3 times each:

I deeply and completely love and accept myself!
I am worthy of the purest love!
I am wanted and loved!
My heart is open to love!
I forgive myself!
I release and let go of all resentment!
I live in harmony and balance with all other beings! I create loving and supportive relationships.

19. COMMUNICATION AFFIRMATIONS:

Affirm and repeat 3 times each:

I am sacred, worthy, and valuable!
I am fulfilled and strong!

I am loved and honored by my words, deeds, and actions!
I choose to be open, clear, and honest in my communication!
I speak my truth with authenticity!
I easily communicate my feelings and emotions!
I am expressing myself with clear intent!
I express my love and honesty each time I speak!

20. RESPONSIBILITY AFFIRMATIONS:

Affirm and repeat 3 times each:

I am responsible!
I take all responsibility completely and fully!
I will not place blame!
I will convert blame to power!
I build my personal power daily!
I gloriously respond with my God ability!
I receive fully!

21. EMPOWERMENT AFFIRMATIONS:

Affirm and repeat 3 times each:

I pour into me daily!
I pour into me to honor all my relations!
I am successful!
All my relations are successful when I am successful!
I deserve the highest and wisest!
When I win, all my relations win!

22. INNER VOICE POWER CHARGE AFFIRMATION:

At the beginning of Arit 6, you created a personal Inner Voice Power Charge Affirmation.

- Take a few moments to affirm yourself daily.
- Affirm yourself in the morning when you rise and in the night before you fall into slumber.

- Both in the morning and in the night, repeat your Inner Voice Power Charge Affirmation to yourself 3 times: 1 time for your mind, 1 time for your body, and 1 time for your spirit.

23. CROWN AFFIRMATIONS:

Affirm and repeat 3 times each:

I am Divine!
I am enlightened!
I am love and light!
I am one with the universe!
I accept and receive divine knowledge!
My spiritual insight is clear!
I see the divine light in everyone!

24. PROTECTION AFFIRMATIONS:

Affirm and repeat 3 times each:

I exercise emotional self-protection with ease!
I am always divinely protected under all circumstances!
I am divinely protected, guided, and strengthened daily!
I live in a divine circle of protection!
I am confident that I am always protected by the Creator!
I am content and protected during my travels always!
I am always surrounded by the Creator's protective light!
I am always shielded from harm!
I always focus on clarity and psychic protection!
I am protected because of my Affirmation Confirmations!
All my friends and family are divinely protected!

25. GRATITUDE AFFIRMATIONS:

Affirm and repeat 3 times each:

I am gloriously grateful right here, right now!

I am grateful that I have my breath!
I am grateful to be alive!
I receive this glorious day!
I am grateful for this moment!

26. ANCESTOR AFFIRMATIONS:

Affirm and repeat 3 times each:

I am my ancestors' prayers answered!
My ancestors smile upon me!
My ancestors wash away my pain!

27. POWER AFFIRMATIONS:

Affirm and repeat 3 times each:

I am the master of this very moment!
I am the word living made manifest in holy flesh!
The holy word is in my eyes, limbs, organs, and cells!
I claim my highest ascension now!
I am more powerful, more mighty!

NUTRITION KITCHEN PHARMACY

NOTE: There are 4 levels of Nutrition Kitchen Pharmacy. Throughout your 12-week Wellness Warrior journey from Arit 1 to Arit 12, refer to the appropriate Nutrition Kitchen Pharmacy level.

NUTRITION KITCHEN PHARMACY LEVEL 1
BEGINNER—FLEXITARIAN OR VEGETARIAN

WEEK 1—THE FAMILY MAN
WEEK 2—THE SENSUAL MAN
WEEK 3—THE TRANSFORMATION MAN

Consume vegetable protein as well as organic chicken and unshelled fish. Incorporate beans, peas, sprouts, and lentils into your diet. Omit all other flesh foods (beef, pork, lamb, turkey, goat, etc.). Consume more fresh fruits, vegetables, and other whole grains.

Pre-Breakfast (Liquid)	Kidney-Liver Flush: Juice of 1 lemon, 1 pinch cayenne pepper (if no HBP), 1–2 Tbsp Inner-Colon Ease, 8 oz warm water w/1–2 garlic cloves or 12 drops of kyolic Tool: Blender
Liquid Breakfast 7:00	Master Herbal Tea or Man's Life Tea *(Alternate every 7 days)* 8–12 oz orange juice w/1–2 Tbsp Green Life in 12–16 oz distilled water
Solid Breakfast 7:30	*30-min break between eating & drinking for optimal digestion of meal* 1–2 mangos or 1 whole cantaloupe *Optional: whole-grain cereal with almond or sesame milk
Liquid Lunch 12:00	Juice: ½ cup kale, ½ cup string beans, ½ cup cabbage Add 1–2 Tbsp Green Life Formula or 1 oz wheatgrass + 8–12 oz water Tool: Juicer *30-min break between eating & drinking for optimal digestion of meal*
Solid Lunch 12:30	50% live greens salad: asparagus w/dandelion greens 30% steamed veggies: mustard greens w/pearl onions or vegetable broth/soup 10%—20% starch: soaked couscous w/sunflower seeds & spike seasonings 10%—20% protein: BBQ or baked organic chicken (remove skin) *Eat animal protein midday only or steam unshelled fish.*
Liquid Dinner 6:00	Repeat vegetable juice from lunch, and add 1–2 Tbsp Green Life + 8 oz water

Solid Dinner 6:30	50% live greens salad: escarole, kale w/red pepper 30% steamed veggies: curry cauliflower 10%—20% starch: millet 10%—20% vegan protein *When the sun goes down, do not eat proteins or starches. Eat only fruits & salads.*

NUTRITION KITCHEN PHARMACY LEVEL 2

INTERMEDIATE—VEGETARIAN

WEEK 4—THE LOVER MAN

WEEK 5—THE COMMUNICATIVE MAN

WEEK 6—THE INTUITIVE MAN

Consume only vegetarian foods. Omit all flesh foods (seafood, beef, pork, lamb, turkey, goat, etc.). Fresh vegetable intake includes 50%—75% live food and 25%—50% steamed to retain as much of the live enzymes and oxygen as possible.

Pre-Breakfast (Liquid)	Kidney-Liver Flush: Juice of 1 lemon, 1 pinch cayenne pepper (if no HBP), 1–2 Tbsp Inner-Colon Ease, 8 oz warm water w/1–2 garlic cloves or 12 drops kyolic Tool: Blender
Liquid Breakfast 7:00	Blue- & Blackberry juice w/1–2 Tbsp Green Life Formula, Master Herbal Tea, or Man's Life Tea
Solid Breakfast 7:30	Blueberries w/blended pears sprinkled w/coconut Blueberries w/blue corn cereal & almond milk *30-minute break between eating & drinking*
Liquid Lunch 12:00	Juice: 2 stalks celery, ½ cup broccoli, ½ cup chard Add 1–2 Tbsp Green Life Formula Tool: Juicer

Solid Lunch 12:30	50% salad w/ live greens: romaine lettuce w/shredded broccoli 30% steamed veggies: zucchini 10%—20% starch: soaked couscous w/sunflower seeds & spike seasonings 10%—20% protein: chickpea curry
Liquid Dinner 6:00	2–4 oz wheatgrass or 1–2 Tbsp Green Life, with 12–16 oz water
Solid Dinner 6:30	50% salad w/ live greens: salad of choice 30% steamed veggies: steamed veggies of choice 10%—20% starch: whole-grain brown rice 10%—20% protein: black bean soup

NUTRITION KITCHEN PHARMACY LEVEL 3
ADVANCED—VEGAN (RAW)
BEGINNING OF 21-DAY RAW FAST

WEEK 7—THE HUMANITARIAN MAN

WEEK 8—THE ILLUMINATED MAN

WEEK 9—THE HARMONIZING MAN

Consume 100% live uncooked food. Live foods include organic live proteins (sprouted beans, raw soaked nuts and seeds, avocados), salads, live soups, uncooked grains such as couscous, tabouli, bulgur wheat, etc. Consume whole or juiced fresh fruits and vegetables. Drink daily warm water (8 oz glasses), 5 cups Master Herbal Tea, and 8 oz of Kidney-Liver Flush.

Pre-Breakfast (Liquid)	Kidney-Liver Flush: Juice of 1 lemon, 1 pinch cayenne pepper (if no HBP), 1–2 Tbsp Inner-Colon Ease, 8 oz warm water w/1–2 garlic cloves or 12 drops kyolic Tool: Blender
Liquid Breakfast 7:00	8 oz unsweetened cranberry juice w/1–2 Tbsp Green Life Master Herbal Tea or Man's Life Tea *30-minute break between eating & drinking*

Solid Breakfast 7:30	Pears w/blueberries, strawberries, or raspberries: Blend to a sauce or slice fruit Pumpkin seeds: soak ½ cup pumpkin seeds for the prostate
Liquid Lunch 12:00	Blood-Restorer Juice: ½ cup kale, ½ cup chard, 1–2 red radishes, ¼ cup ginger root, & ½ beet Stir in 1–2 Tbsp Green Life upon completion Tool: Juicer
Solid Lunch 12:30	50% salad w/live greens: grated beets & red peppers 30% steamed veggies: 1 cup raw okra with olive oil & spike seasonings 10%—20% starch: mock tuna wrapped in lettuce or seaweed 10%—20% protein: ½ cup broccoli sprouts or mung beans over salad
Liquid Dinner 6:00	Repeat Blood-Restorer Juice from lunch. Add 1–2 Tbsp Green Life.
Solid Dinner 6:30	50% salad w/live greens: spinach salad w/mung beans 30% steamed veggies: steamed or live okra 10%—20% starch: steamed couscous 10%—20% protein: 2 Tbsp coconut aminos over grain or ½ avocado

NUTRITION KITCHEN PHARMACY LEVEL 4
ADVANCED—WHOLE FOOD HEALING JUICE FAST

WEEK 10—THE NATURE MAN

WEEK 11—THE ALCHEMIST MAN

WEEK 12—THE SELF-MASTERY MAN

Consume 100% organic liquid meals only. This cleanse consists of 2 vegetable juice meals for rejuvenation and 1 fruit juice meal for detoxification daily. Additionally, there is a daily intake of ½ gallon warm water (8 oz glasses), 5 cups Master Herbal Tea, and 8 oz of Kidney-Liver Flush.

Pre-Breakfast (Liquid)	Kidney-Liver Flush: Juice of 1 lemon, 1 pinch cayenne pepper (if no HBP), 1–2 Tbsp Inner-Colon Ease, 8 oz warm water w/1–2 garlic cloves or 12 drops kyolic Tool: Blender
Liquid Breakfast 7:00	8 oz unsweetened cranberry juice w/1–2 Tbsp Green Life Master Herbal Tea or Man's Life Tea
Liquid Breakfast 12:00	2–4 oz wheatgrass w/12–16 oz distilled water OR Juice: ½ cup beets; ½ cup kale; ½ cup chard Stir in 1–2 Tbsp Green Life upon completion Tool: Juicer
Liquid Dinner 6:00	Juice: ¼ cup spinach or 1–2 Tbsp Green Life in 12–16 oz pure water Tool: Juicer

WEEKLY CHECK-UP CHART

(SAMPLE)

NOTE: Throughout your 12-week Wellness Warrior journey, it is important to remind yourself of daily assignments. When you complete them, it is important to check them off so you can see your progress toward Optimal Wellness.

- Replicate this MHT WEEKLY CHECK-UP CHART (or create your own).
- You will need 12 charts, 1 for each week of your 12-week Wellness Warrior journey.
- Date each chart.

SUNRISE WELLNESS	Day 1	Day 2	Day 3	Day 4	Day 5	Day 6	Day 7
Spiritual Observances: Recite/Reflect on Affirmations from Antiquity, do altar work and journaling							
Kidney Liver Flush: Drink the juice of 1 lemon and 16 oz warm water with 2 tbsp of Colon Ease							
Liquid Breakfast: Drink Master Herbal Formula; have 8 oz fresh juice with 8 oz water + 1–2 Tbsp of Green Life or Supa Mega Greens							
Solid Breakfast: Fresh fruit of choice (mangos, pears, blueberries)							
Complete MHT Daily Workout							

MIDDAY WELLNESS (Lunch)	**Day 1**	**Day 2**	**Day 3**	**Day 4**	**Day 5**	**Day 6**	**Day 7**
Midday Affirmations							
Inversion for 10 minutes							
Liquid Lunch: Green Life (8–16 oz fresh juice or water with 1–2 Tbsp of Green Life)							
Solid Green Power Lunch (salad/ steamed vegetables/ whole grains/protein, e.g., beans, lentils)							
Flexitarian Lunch: steamed fish as protein with vegetables and whole grains							

SUNSET WELLNESS (Dinner)	Day 1	Day 2	Day 3	Day 4	Day 5	Day 6	Day 7
Sunset Affirmations							
Liquid Dinner: 8–16 oz vegetable juice and water with 1–2 tbsp Green Life Nutritional Formula or Supa Mega Greens							
Green Power Dinner (salad/steamed vegetables/whole grains/protein, e.g., beans, peas, lentils)							
Flexitarian Dinner: steamed fish as protein with vegetables and whole grains							
Men's Life or Master Herbal Tonic Directions: Add 6 tbsp to 4 oz of boiling water and let steep for 1 hr (off the stove). Drink in the a.m. (Rotate every 7 days.)							

SUNSET WELLNESS (Dinner, continued)	**Day 1**	**Day 2**	**Day 3**	**Day 4**	**Day 5**	**Day 6**	**Day 7**
Sunset Affirmations							
Internal Cleansing: Take 3 Herbal Laxative Tablets before bed							
Detox Bath: Fill a tub with warm water and add 1–2 lbs Epsom salt Soak for 30 minutes							
Zone Body Massage: Body, face, and hands							
Clay Poultice: Apply clay overnight to any body part in need							

Journaling is one of your daily assignments. Replicate the sample below (or create your own journal pages). Be sure to date each journal entry. Try to journal *at least* once a week; even better, once a day.

VISION QUEST JOURNAL PAGE

RISE | SHINE | LISTEN | RECEIVE | ACTIVATE

Date: ______________________________

THE POWER TO HEAL IS WITHIN

CHAPTER **6**

The First 7 Arit States of Man

LIST OF THE FIRST 7 ARIT STATES OF MAN

ARIT STATE 1:
The Family Man of Unity and Wealth

ARIT STATE 2:
The Sensual Man of Heightened Sensitivity

ARIT STATE 3:
The Transformation Man of Renewal

ARIT STATE 4:
The Lover Man of Harmony

ARIT STATE 5:
The Communication Man of Connectivity and Creativity

ARIT STATE 6:
The Intuitive Man of Clear Vision

ARIT STATE 7:
The Universal Humanitarian Man

ARIT 1: THE FAMILY MAN OF UNITY AND WEALTH

> "I come into being from unformed matter. Make me always prosperous. Triumphantly gather my bones and collect my limbs."
>
> —THE PAPYRUS OF ANI

OPENING THE WAY:

The Family Man represents unity. Unity represents harmony. Harmony creates abundance. Abundance penetrates your deepest inner self to receive from the Creator what is needed in the present moment. Poverty is the result of discord and being out of alignment with the Creator and with yourself. Discord exists when the mind, body, and spirit are not unified and not in harmonious balance.

For one to be the Family Man, he must establish an inner state of unity with his mind, body, and spirit. The Family Man's initial focus is with himself, constructing abundance from within. The building and creating start with him first on a micro level, pouring into the source which is himself with an abundance mindset. Pouring abundance into his Mind, Body, and Spirit.

Strengthening his inner self daily on a subconscious level through the cultivation of personal power and the knowledge that everything begins with him. Affirming himself daily with creative attributes that empower and strengthen is key to showing up as his most fully expressed self. Prioritizing himself and being disciplined with his self-mastery is a salute to his absolute value in order to be fully charged and activated to execute his mission and obligations.

Shaping and molding himself into his most authentic and truthful self is creating a man of his highest value and wisest self. Going within daily and tackling the challenging inner work to become whole strengthens himself to provide for his family with unity and wealth.

As a man unifies his inner self, his family reflects his inner harmony. The Family Man makes every possible effort to secure his own as well as his family's survival with food, clothing, and shelter. The Family Man's world revolves around building family by nurturing and nourishing himself and his family through communication and cultivation of himself and his family.

The Family Man is in alignment with the knowledge that family is the foundation and the root of success. Once he can build abundance within himself, the Family Man is able to build material abundance in order to stabilize the unity and growth of the family through balance and self-mastery. To manifest and acquire a strong family, the Family Man must possess creativity, vision, and an unwavering balanced inner power, inspiring and empowering himself and his family throughout his journey.

The Family Man dwells in the root coccygeal power center that houses the skin, legs, feet, muscular system, and bones. More than 17 million men have doctor-diagnosed arthritis. Half of Americans with arthritis don't think anything can be done to help them. More than 16 million non-Hispanic Blacks report doctor-diagnosed arthritis.

AFFIRM AND FORGIVE

Wellness Salute, Beloved Brother! Man Heal Thyself Wellness Warrior is a Fraternity of Wellness, a fellowship of brothers who use holistic practices, rituals, traditions, and celebrations to encourage and to hold each other accountable. You are part of this community, an integral member of this brotherhood.

By pledging daily through your actions of commitment to a holistic lifestyle, you are choosing to love and to accept yourself unconditionally. You are choosing to prioritize your self-care by committing to pouring into yourself mentally, emotionally, spiritually, and physically. You are pledging to create the space and time to affirm and to forgive.

A blockage is an obstruction that makes movement or flow difficult or impossible. A blockage is a barrier that is being restrictive and stagnant. Blockages may be emotional, relating to your heart; psychological, relating to your mind; spiritual, relating to your relationship with the Most High; energetic, relating to your Energy System; environmental, relating to your surroundings. Blockages may be connected to people, places, or things. Blockages may be stress-induced, anxiety-induced, fear-induced, belief-induced. Blockages may be caused by limited thinking, critical thinking, negative self-talk. A blockage may be the result of insecurities, the need for control, avoidance, self-imposed limitations, repetitive patterns, resistance to change, or communication breakdown.

Finding a way to overcome your blockages enables you to grow as a person instead of staying stagnant and repeating unhealthy and toxic patterns. One such way to overcome blockages is to acknowledge your block or blocks. This acknowledgment can be achieved through daily affirmations. By affirming yourself, you move yourself into a positive, heightened space that opens a spiritual portal to higher consciousness.

Being a Black Man, let alone a Man in this society, you have the responsibility to affirm yourself in a world that does not affirm you. Maybe you have navigated between family dysfunction and societal dysfunction, warping your self-value and how you see yourself. Affirming yourself daily throughout your self-development journey is important and imperative to strengthening your sense of who you are and how you value yourself. To confirm your affirmation is to review the action steps taken to achieve your daily Wellness Goals. Affirmations are the pathway to create and to enter your Accountability Matrix.

The act of affirming yourself in the present tense and confirming yourself strengthens your divine attributes of self-development, healing, restoration, self-praise, self-visualization, forgiveness, and gratitude.

To affirm is to state as a fact, to assert strongly and publicly, and to offer emotional support or encouragement. Affirmation is the action or process of affirming something or being affirmed. Dear Brother, the time for action is now! So, what are you affirming about yourself? What is your Affirmation Confirmation to yourself?

Affirmation Confirmation is not about your mother affirming you, your father affirming you, or society affirming you. You, yourself, have to be the affirmation. As a Black Man, as a Man, you must affirm yourself with the power and intensity to awaken yourself to the now, to the present.

To affirm yourself is to strengthen yourself in the present into the highest vision of yourself. Affirmation Confirmations are pledges to yourself. Affirmation Confirmations are a way to create a current paradigm of your actions to give you high results to affirm who you are. Affirmation Confirmations are personal tools for you to remember who you are and what you are capable of achieving and accomplishing with strength, courage, power, and resilience. So, dear Brother, empower yourself through your words.

Another way to reclaim your power, dear Brother, is to identify your blockages through the act of forgiveness—forgiving yourself and forgiving others. Forgiveness is an opportunity to release self-judgment. Forgiveness is an act of liberation and freedom for yourself.

When you are unable to affirm yourself daily, which is an act of reminding yourself who you really are—the highest version of yourself—you have the possibility of staying blocked in a perpetual space of guilt and shame. Some of the blockages that you face when you forget to affirm yourself can often be around guilt and the inability to forgive.

A Man often has the habit of not letting things go. You may move on, but you don't actually let that thing go. You hold on to that disappointment, shame, guilt, frustration, and blame. Sometimes you are clinging to that thing from when you were 3 years old, 5 years old, 15 years old, 22 years old. By allowing things to fester within, those things tend to build up and cause blockages in the colon of your life.

Addressing your blockages may be one of the most challenging aspects of your Man Heal Thyself Wellness Warrior journey. Know that you are not judged for your blockages. Know that you are greater than any of your blockages. The courage of sharing your blockages will be affirmed back into you as well as heal millions of Men. Your healing represents millions of Men healing themselves as you become an example of higher consciousness.

BELOVED BROTHER, YOU ARE THE WORD MADE MANIFEST IN FLESH!

"We must develop and maintain the capacity to forgive.

He who is devoid of the power to forgive is devoid of the power to love.

There is some good in the worst of us and some evil in the best of us.

When we discover this, we are less prone to hate our enemies."

—MARTIN LUTHER KING JR.

American Baptist Minister and Activist

AFFIRM AND FORGIVE ASSIGNMENT:

PART 1: AFFIRMATION CONFIRMATION

- Create your own personal Affirmation Confirmation, which will be your daily mantra to spell you out of your lower self into your higher consciousness. Your Affirmation Confirmation is your passcode for reentry into Divine Order.
  - — What can you say to yourself to snap yourself out of being complacent, limited, and down on yourself?
  - — What words of power do you need to tell yourself daily to stand mighty and bold in your sovereignty?
  - — Who are you at your essence when ego, insecurities, and self-doubts are released?
- Write down 2 lines/sentences to affirm yourself.

Examples:

— I, SupaNova Slom, affirm all day and every day, to be accountable to my highest and wisest self to nourish myself so that I can continue to serve humanity at the highest level.

— I, Halleluyah Walcott, am imbued with the power of the universe. I am the living proof of something higher existing on this physical plane.

PRACTICE:

— Take a few moments to affirm yourself daily.

— Affirm yourself in the morning when you rise and in the night before you fall into slumber.

— Both in the morning and in the night, repeat your Affirmation Confirmation to yourself 3 times: 1 time for your mind, 1 time for your body, and 1 time for you.

PART 2: LETTER OF APOLOGY TO YOURSELF

- Write a letter of apology to yourself for releasing yourself of your past transgressions, whether against yourself or others. Let go of actions, deeds, and things that you are not proud of. Release your history along with past hurts and pains that you might be holding on to. Let go of malthoughts that are preventing you from moving forward.

PART 3: IDENTIFYING BLOCKAGES AND RELEASING SELF-JUDGMENT

- For this exercise, identify and write down 3 to 5 blocks that you feel you need to overcome. Once you identify and overcome these blocks, there will be no limits to how you will grow and develop, no limits to what you will achieve. The abundance will be flowing to, around, and from you.
  - — What blocks have been getting in your way?
  - — What blocks have been holding you back in your self-development?
  - — What blocks have you not been able to let go of?
  - — What people? What places? What things?
  - — What has kept you stagnant and restricted in ways that have prevented you from healing and moving forward? Maybe it's money, emotional wounds, traumas.
  - — What have you allowed to become part of your being and reality that no longer suits you?

PART 4: PRAYER OF FORGIVENESS

- Create your own personal Prayer of Forgiveness.
- Write down 3 to 5 lines/sentences to yourself related to anything that you feel you need to forgive yourself for.
- What is your act of forgiveness to yourself? What are you forgiving yourself for?

- Do you need to forgive yourself for being hard on yourself, not listening or not trusting yourself? Do you need to forgive yourself for not having the courage you needed to have in certain relationships, certain tasks? Do you need to forgive yourself for not achieving your wellness goals? Do you need to forgive yourself for your food choices? What do you feel you have dropped the ball with?
- You want your Prayer of Forgiveness to hold yourself accountable while releasing self-judgment and self-criticism.

Remember: As a Man, when you forgive yourself, you are representing millions of men forgiving and healing themselves.

Examples:

— I, SupaNova Slom, forgive myself for not trusting my intuition. I forgive myself for not always keeping discipline with my daily warrior tasks and drills. With this forgiveness, I reclaim and reaffirm my commitment.

— I, Halleluyah Walcott, forgive myself for my lack of discipline at times. I forgive myself for the self-imposed pressures of perfection that cause inaction and inhibit me from achieving my goals. With this forgiveness, I am renewed and revitalized.

PRACTICE:

— Take a few moments to say your Prayer of Forgiveness at least once a day.

ARIT 1: THE FAMILY MAN DAILY SPIRITUAL OBSERVANCES

ARIT POWER CENTER: Coccygeal Root, Skin, Legs, Feet, Muscles, and Bones
ARIT COLOR: Red

1. **THE SPIRITUAL BATH**

2. **AROMATHERAPY**

3. **YOUR ALTAR**

4. **ARIT 1 AFFIRMATION:**

   "I come into being
   From unformed matter.
   Make me always prosperous
   Triumphantly gather my bones
   And collect my limbs."
   —*The Papyrus of Ani*

5. **LIBATION**

6. **MAN HEAL THYSELF WELLNESS WARRIOR PRAYER**

7. **COCCYGEAL ROOT EMPOWERMENT AND DETOXIFICATION AFFIRMATION—ARIT 1:**

   My life is abundantly full and overflowing with greatness. May I be empowered to overcome financial lack. May I attract and build prosperity in all ways of my life. May my financial abundance flow like a river to and from me. May I create work that reflects my purpose. May I not abuse myself. May I not abuse my family.

   May I not be abused by my family. May I work with my family to build a powerful, self-sustaining unit that supplies all our needs. May I, as a Man, bring to my family unity, power, and strength so that we not only survive but that we, as a family, thrive. Today, I attract not poverty but wealth. I vibrate at the frequency of Skhm, which represents power and vitality. As I heal, may I bring power and vitality to my family. May my family honor and care for me in return.

8. **CHANT (HESI)**
9. **FIRE BREATHS**
10. **HEALING STONE MEDITATION AND VISUALIZATION**
11. **HERBAL TONICS**
12. **WELLNESS WARRIOR JOURNAL WRITING**
13. **AFFIRMATION CONFIRMATION**
14. **PRAYER OF FORGIVENESS**
15. **PROBLEM-SOLVER AFFIRMATIONS**
16. **VALUE AND POWER AFFIRMATIONS**
17. **EXERCISE: COMPLETE YOUR WORKOUT FROM THE MAN HEAL THYSELF 12-WEEK WORKOUT PLAN**

HEALING THE WOUNDED CHILD

FROM A HURT BOY TO A MAN IN HEALING

Childhood experiences shape our lives in profound ways, and for some, those experiences are marked by pain and hurt. The wounded child, a metaphorical representation of the inner child wounded by emotional scars, carries these wounds into adulthood. However, with time, self-reflection, and a commitment to healing, a hurt boy can transform into a resilient man—often through the following stages:

1. Acknowledging the Wounds: The first step in healing the wounded child is acknowledging the wounds and their impact. It requires confronting the pain, traumas, and unresolved emotions from the past. Revisit the first Arit—The Family Man of Unity and Wealth. Revisit the steps of the assignment: the letter of apology to yourself, identifying blockages and releasing self-judgment, and saying the prayer for forgiveness. Reviewing these exercises may prompt you to address any unhealed wounds. This recognition allows the hurt boy to begin understanding the wounds and their influence on his behavior, relationships, and self-perception.
2. Reconnecting with the Inner Child: Reconnecting with the wounded inner child is a crucial aspect of healing. It involves creating a safe space for the hurt boy to express his emotions, fears, and unmet needs. Your training in the beginning of this text has prepared the young boy inner child to be much more forgiving, resilient, and able to apply self-care. By acknowledging and embracing the inner child in this way, a wounded boy can begin nurturing and soothing the pain within.
3. Seeking Support: Healing the wounded child is not a journey that one must undertake alone. Seeking support from trusted

individuals, such as therapists, support groups, or loved ones, can provide invaluable guidance and encouragement. These individuals can offer empathy, validation, and a safe space for the hurt boy to share his experiences. Through this support network, the wounded child can find strength, validation, and a sense of belonging.

4. Unlearning negative patterns is a transformative process that begins with awareness and self-reflection. First, the individual must recognize and acknowledge the negative behaviors or thought patterns influenced by their wounded inner child. This can be achieved through therapy, where guided sessions help uncover deeply rooted issues. Next, journaling or engaging in mindfulness practices can facilitate self-discovery, allowing one to explore the feelings and triggers associated with negative patterns. The third step involves challenging negative beliefs by questioning their validity and replacing them with positive affirmations. Seeking support from trusted friends or support groups can provide encouragement and accountability. Finally, consistently practicing healthier alternatives—such as positive self-talk, setting boundaries, and engaging in self-care—helps reinforce new habits and fosters emotional resilience. With patience and persistence, individuals can gradually shift their mindset and cultivate a more positive, fulfilling life.
5. Cultivating Self-Compassion and Self-Love: The commitment to personal growth supported by a therapist or supportive network is key to aiding the wounded child in cultivating a new and healthy sense of self-compassion and self-love. The hurt boy must learn to treat himself with kindness, empathy, and understanding. Again, refer to the exercises and assignments in Arit 1 to reacquaint the Extended Warrior with the introduction to techniques and practices for developing self-awareness and self-care as expanded upon throughout the text. By de-

veloping a nurturing relationship with oneself, the wounded child can begin to heal the emotional wounds and rebuild a positive self-image.

As the healing journey progresses, the hurt boy can transform into a man in healing, marked by growth and resilience. The wounds of the past become a source of wisdom and strength rather than a source of pain. By acknowledging the wounds, reconnecting with the inner child, seeking support, unlearning negative patterns, cultivating self-compassion, and embracing growth, a hurt boy can evolve into a resilient man in healing. This journey is not without its challenges, but the rewards are immense—freedom from the past, inner peace, and a renewed sense of self.

UNLOCKING SACRED UNION

(THE HARMONY OF THE DIVINE MASCULINE AND DIVINE FEMININE)

Before discussing the concept of the harmony of the Divine Masculine and Divine Feminine, we must acknowledge the working definitions of masculine and of feminine and, then, of Divine. Throughout human history, numerous religious, cultural, and political groups have defined the attributes and assigned the roles of women and men according to the say-so in their community. Often, creativity, nurturing, and intuition have been assigned as female principles and attributes. At the same time, men are identified as the providers, the protectors, and the problem-solvers. These energies exist within each person, irrespective of biology, and are essential for a balanced and fulfilling life.

Clarity must be established that the *principles* are not gender specific; the principles are universally present and interchangeable attributes in men and women. The principles are, in fact, tools. Men and women must work on using their tools to heal themselves in order to attain their optimal state of expression and well-being.

The divine masculine and divine feminine are archetypal energies that transcend gender and are present in all individuals. We are born divine. Our divinity is the microcosm of the macrocosmic creation of all life. So, if it is said that the divine masculine represents qualities such as strength, assertiveness, logic, and action, while the divine feminine embodies qualities such as intuition, nurturing, compassion, and receptivity, then the reverse for both is true.

When the divine masculine and divine feminine energies are balanced and integrated within an individual, an extraordinary transformation occurs. The harmonious interplay between the active and receptive forces yields a state of wholeness and inner peace. It empowers individuals to embrace their unique strengths and vulnerabilities, leading to personal growth and self-realization.

The sacred union extends beyond the individual level and has a profound impact on relationships. When two individuals embody the harmonious balance of the divine masculine and divine feminine, their connection becomes a sacred gift. In such relationships, mutual respect, deep understanding, and unconditional love flourish. The synergy of these energies creates a dynamic partnership, where each person supports and uplifts the other, fostering growth and spiritual evolution.

The sacred union embodies the balance, synergy, and interconnectedness between the masculine and feminine energies within us and the world around us, manifesting as a sacred gift that continuously enriches our lives.

As more individuals awaken to the importance of embracing both their masculine and feminine aspects, societal structures can begin to shift. The rigid gender roles and stereotypes that have long constrained human potential start to dissolve, allowing for a more inclusive and egalitarian society. This transformation fosters collaboration, empathy, and respect among all individuals, leading to a harmonious coexistence.

In Ma'at (Harmony, Balance)

ARIT 2: THE SENSUAL MAN OF HEIGHTENED SENSITIVITY

"Purification is on this day of my birth.
I am purified. My phallus is of divinity."
—THE PAPYRUS OF ANI

OPENING THE WAY:

The Sensual Man is activated, authentic, and awakened with heightened senses and emotions. He welcomes what lies beneath the surface, embracing the soul, the heart, and the mind. He understands the power of being present and the importance of being seen and recognized on a deep and attentive level.

The Sensual Man is in tune with all his senses—his visual sight, his inner sight, his taste, his smell, and his touch—and is thus alive and aware of self and of the woman in his life and of life in general. He knows what it means to be vulnerable and is not afraid to show who he is. His sensitivity creates paths to deeper connections and opens doors of intimacy.

The Sensual Man values himself and those around him. He is resilient and courageous, tender and commanding. He pays attention to detail, focusing on the journey and the process. The Sensual Man sees life as an opportunity to risk, to feel, to experience, and to love. He is the embodiment of a full and passionate life, as he is in alignment with self through balance and harmony. He is joyful, playful, and fun. His inner child beams with delight at the possibilities of discovery through his senses and embraces the newfound treasures.

The Sensual Man is firm in body, steady in disposition, and warm of heart. He will listen attentively, hearing others' thoughts. He will be intimate, sensitive, and connected, paying attention to others' moves. The Sensual Man knows when to be still. He also knows when and how to approach.

The Sensual Man acknowledges both the divine masculine and divine feminine within him. He embraces this powerful force of masculine and feminine energies within him to strengthen and nourish his spirit. He accesses this polarity within him as the foundation for his creative force and releases his ego. The Sensual Man is in harmony with his masculine and feminine balance, his left and right brain, and his consciousness.

The Sensual Man's genitals are in their prime. With a total vibrant flow of blood and oxygen derived from a holistic wellness plant-based lifestyle, the Sensual Man maintains a potent, sensual, sexual life. With his words and actions, the Sensual Man conceives and manifests healthy visions, creations, children, and worlds.

IDENTIFY AND TRANSFORM:

Wellness Salute, Beloved Brother! Mindfulness daily is the highest attribute that activates your personal Godhead through your personal values, love, and gratitude. When you activate your holistic protocols daily, you strengthen your alpha Man Heal Thyself Wellness Warrior power. You are choosing the highest vibrational value, which activates high-vibrational mind, body, and spirit protocols for your optimal wellness. For example, when interacting with your partner, having a clear mind, body, and spirit is critical.

When your interaction is clouded and distorted, you signal pain and confusion. The womb is a chamber, a sacred portal of time and space, that holds and cultivates whatever is placed within it. As a result, you must prepare your energy force, vibration, vitality, and thoughts with the highest and cleanest version of yourself before sexual transference. The womb will birth your highest or lowest vibration, your God cells or your Devil seeds. You are what you feed your mind, body, and spirit daily. So, if you are not affirming yourself daily and prioritizing self-care, then you leave yourself open to attack from your low-vibrational ego. In turn, you are making yourself a soft target for external attacks.

When you are forgetful or out of harmony and balance with your daily flow of wellness, you open a portal of low-vibrational living that contaminates your ability to be abundant, whole, and virile. By opening a portal of low-vibrational living, you are activating a beta cadence that removes your Godhead and triggers the "God Damn Fool."

As a man, there are times when you may be dimming your own light by not using your voice or not expressing your real emotions and feelings. In these moments, you may be emotionally blocked, as you may not want to open up and be vulnerable out of fear, rejection, or past traumas. You might find it easier to create a wall by being cold and standoffish to others, though behind your self-imposed wall, you may yearn for connection, intimacy, sensuality, and vulnerability.

As a Man Heal Thyself Wellness Warrior, your commitment to yourself and to your self-care is to pour into yourself daily. By claiming your light, you are standing in your power and your truth, declaring your voice and embracing your emotions and feelings. You are taking ownership of all aspects of who you are and making the choice to release your emotional blockages. You are making the choice to identify what needs healing within you by challenging yourself to transform. As an alpha man, you seek to problem-solve within yourself as well as within the world.

Dear Brother, real power and strength are found in vulnerability. Real power and strength are found in acknowledging your emotions and feelings. Real power and strength are found in using your voice to express who you really are without allowing fear, rejection, or past traumas to control and to inhibit you. Real power and strength are found in your ability to stand up to the pervasive male toxicity in Western culture.

Real power and strength are found in living a balanced, harmonious, high-vibrational life that recognizes that both the divine masculine and divine feminine exist simultaneously within all.

To serve your mate, family, friends, community, society, and the world, you must serve yourself as the God-Man daily. The union of the Creator and yourself is the most critical union, for all that you are begins with the Great One. To be inside the Creator, to be fully aware of the Creator's presence within you, and to be guided by the Most High, you must first love yourself as the Creator loves you. When you truly love yourself, you become one with the divine. It is then that the Creator can enter your house and all your unions will be blessed.

Everyone has at least three or more active aspects or personalities within themselves. Each of these personalities develops within divine time to aid growth and development. To be effective, these various parts within you must come into harmonious union and work together for the greater good. For example, one self-protects, another inspires, a third is brilliant, and yet another is sensual and sensitive. The male and female aspects within everyone must come together with love. These complementary, yet opposite facets of the divine masculine and divine feminine must unite into one team, one entity with the strength necessary to ultimately give you all that is needed for your journey through life.

Once the two forces of male and female come together in complete harmony, Heaven and Earth become one. By being a part of a Fraternity of Wellness, you are committing to yourself, to the Creator, and to the planet the process of healing yourself. You are choosing to open your heart to the love and the sensitivities within you and others. You are choosing to develop harmony first within yourself, balancing your own inner masculine and feminine forces. Once you establish a balanced state, all answers will reveal themselves to your new consciousness—a new perspective, a whole new way of being.

BELOVED BROTHER, YOU ARE THE MIGHTY AND VICTORIOUS PROBLEM-SOLVER!

> "Change will not come if we wait for some other person or some other time.
> We are the ones we've been waiting for.
> We are the change that we seek."
>
> —BARACK OBAMA
>
> *44th President of the United States*

IDENTIFY AND TRANSFORM ASSIGNMENT:

PART 1: MOST IMPACTED (Smile)

- Identify 3 people who had the most profound impact on you intimately.
  - Intimately could be a committed relationship, a one-night stand, etc.
- Write down these 3 names.
- Next to each person's name, write 1 power word that describes this person, a power word that makes you think of that person, or a power word that resonates with you about the feeling you experienced with this person.

PART 2: MOST DISAPPOINTED (Frown)

- Identify 3 people who broke your heart and/or your trust.
- Who has most disappointed you?
- Write down these 3 names.
- Next to each person's name, write a short sentence or a few words that describe what happened.
  - How was your heart broken? How was your trust broken? How were you disappointed? What was the trigger?

PART 3: RELEASING EMOTIONAL BLOCKS

- Identify and write down 3 to 5 emotional blocks that have held you back and/or prevented you from moving forward and/or going deeper in your relationships. Go as deep as you can.
  - Why have you been emotionally blocked in your relationships?
  - Why do you not want to open up and be vulnerable in your relationships?
  - Why do you become cold and distant?
  - Why is it easier to be cold and distant than vulnerable?

— Why do you find it challenging to acknowledge and to express your emotions and feelings in relationships?
— What childhood events and traumas have impacted you and caused you to be closed off emotionally?
— What events and traumas in your life have impacted you and caused you to be closed off emotionally?
— What fears do you have about being vulnerable and expressing your feelings and emotions?
— Why do you long for relationships and community, but when you receive them, you get cold and quiet? Why aren't you willing to pour into your relationships and community?
— Why, when you get what you want, do you shut down emotionally?
— What about the challenge is more thrilling than the prize?
— What are you holding on to and not releasing?
— What is preventing you from having the most complete and powerful relationships with yourself and others?
— What is stopping you from having the most tremendous relationships with your community? With your brothers? With your mother? Father? Family? Mate? Kids?
— How can you tap into the divine feminine that is within you?
— How can you release any toxic masculinity within you?

PART 4: BECOMING A LIBERATED, FULLY EXPRESSED MAN OF LOVE, SENSUALITY, AND HEIGHTENED SENSITIVITY

- Identify and write down 3 to 5 characteristics or attributes that you envision yourself becoming once you claim your liberation as a fully expressed man of love, sensuality, and heightened sensitivity.

- With this exercise, you are setting intentions for the future: how you see yourself expressing your voice, feelings, and emotions in new ways that you have never done before, because now you are healed and unblocked.
- In part 3 of this assignment, you recognized where you were emotionally blocked. For this part, you are visualizing how you see yourself once you have released, transformed, and overcome.
  - What new qualities do you possess as a liberated, fully expressed man of love, sensuality, and heightened sensitivity?
  - How do you define a liberated, fully expressed man of love, sensuality, and heightened sensitivity?
  - How do you embody being a balanced and harmonious alpha male?
  - How do you see yourself expressing your sensitivity and your sensuality?
  - How can you be a better mate who is a liberated, fully expressed man of love, sensuality, and heightened sensitivity? A better son? A better father? A better friend?
  - How can you better express your feelings and emotions?
  - How can you tap into the divine feminine that is within you?
  - How can you release any toxic masculinity within you?
  - What victories are you claiming after releasing your emotional blockages?

ARIT 2: THE SENSUAL MAN DAILY SPIRITUAL OBSERVANCES

ARIT POWER CENTER: SACRAL—PROSTATE, BLADDER, COLON, AND KIDNEYS

ARIT COLOR: ORANGE

1. **THE SPIRITUAL BATH**

2. **AROMATHERAPY**

3. **YOUR ALTAR**

4. **ARIT 2 AFFIRMATION:**

   "Purification is on this day of my birth.
   I am purified.
   My phallus is of divinity."
   —*The Papyrus of Ani*

5. **LIBATION**

6. **MAN HEAL THYSELF WELLNESS WARRIOR PRAYER**

7. **SACRED REPRODUCTIVE EMPOWERMENT AFFIRMATION—ARIT 2:**

   May my sacral center that houses my prostate, colon, bladder, and kidneys function in optimal wellness. May the Divine Healer within me bring forth life and strength in all that I conceive, produce, and generate. May I maintain my youthful sexual and sensual creative life force. May I protect and guide my genitals from toxic thoughts, toxic emotions, toxic substances, and toxic relationships that keep me in a cycle of pain, conflict, constipation, and blockage. May my organs of release, colon, bladder, and kidneys support the purification of my entire anatomy so that I will attract holistically healthy relationships.

8. **CHANT (HESI)**
9. **FIRE BREATHS**
10. **HEALING STONE MEDITATION AND VISUALIZATION**
11. **HERBAL TONIC**
12. **WELLNESS WARRIOR JOURNAL WRITING**
13. **AFFIRMATION CONFIRMATION**
14. **PRAYER OF FORGIVENESS**
15. **PROBLEM-SOLVER AFFIRMATIONS**
16. **VALUE AND POWER AFFIRMATIONS**
17. **EXERCISE: COMPLETE YOUR WORKOUT FROM THE MAN HEAL THYSELF 12-WEEK WORKOUT PLAN**

ARIT 3: THE TRANSFORMATION MAN OF RENEWAL

> "Come forth . . .
> Make the transformation."
>
> —THE PAPYRUS OF ANI

OPENING THE WAY:

The Transformation Man stands in his value and power with confidence and discipline. He takes responsibility for his thoughts, words, actions, and deeds. He views every situation as an opportunity for growth and development, whatever the outcome. The Transformation Man learns from all of life's experiences as he understands that life is filled with victories, which include both wins and lessons.

The Transformation Man ingests his experiences through his mind, body, and spirit, absorbing life, while maintaining balance of health, mind, and strength. As his mind, body, and spirit process his experiences, the Transformation Man is living and digesting the experience.

The experiences that are digestible are part of his life force. The digestible experience and the Transformation Man are in alignment; they are growing together in unison until the moment they transcend the other.

The experiences that are indigestible are not part of the essence and core of who he is. The indigestible experience and the Transformation Man are not in alignment. They are not working together in unity and harmony. Instead, the indigestible experiences are hindering the Transformation Man's growth and development and causing him disease.

Yet the Transformation Man uses his ability to detoxify in order to problem-solve and to find solutions so that the indigestible experiences are released and flushed.

The Transformation Man understands that the process of shifting and changing requires an alignment between the mind, body, and spirit. To elevate spiritually and to ascend to higher frequencies, the mind and body must be cleansed and purified.

The Transformation Man learns from his indigestible experiences through his detoxification. He releases what no longer serves his highest good through a plant-based holistic lifestyle that includes prayer, meditation, visualization, journaling, healing baths, and soul sweats. The Transformation Man learns from every experience, growing, expanding, and ascending. The Transformation Man believes that every life lesson is a blessing.

The Transformation Man metaphysically dwells in the solar plexus, which houses the liver, pancreas, and back. Diabetes is the leading cause of kidney failure in African Americans. The prevalence of diabetes in African Americans is much higher than in white Americans. Thirteen million, or 11.8 percent of all men age 20 years or older have diabetes. Approximately 14.7 percent of all African Americans over 20 years of age (3.7 million) have diabetes. On average, African Americans are twice as likely to have diabetes as white Americans of similar age.

To the men from my clan, who are statistically the most traumatized from 400 years of chattel slavery but who are most elevated as the first healers on Earth, I'm reaching out to you. Those who suffered as a casualty of a stolen legacy and who still suffer from the highest incidences of all disease, including economic starvation, emotional and psychological deprivation, and dietary malnutrition, I'm reaching out to you. To those suffering from the highest incidence of diabetes, high blood pressure, stroke, heart disease, kidney failure, impotence, depression, and premature death, I'm especially reaching out to you to overcome, rise up, and be counted in wellness. For you, the first man of humanity, this is your time.

Man, it's time to make a global shift from using power that destroys to using power that builds. For power that destroys—and in these times especially—creates massive, unrelenting disease, greed, violence, and widespread destruction to nature and to man. This is reflected and expressed through domination, suppression, oppression, and manipulation.

Power that builds is true power. It yields inner harmony, optimal health, and balanced wealth. The Ancient Nile Valley ancestors called this state Ma'at (balance, truth, righteousness, and reciprocity). As one applies the teachings in Man Heal Thyself, one comes into alignment. Man will draw to himself like a magnet abundance in thought, word, and deed—and blossom, he will.

Through man's mental, physical, emotional, social, and sexual elevation, he will shift the current conditions on Earth from toxic people, land, and environment to holistic people who will restore the Earth. "As above, so below; as within, so without." Man's elevation will cause the air and water to purify and the Earth to recover in minerals and mass. Each day that man grows in wellness, he will blossom and shift from an impotent, confused, weak, unsure, ineffective man to a potent, empowered, healthy, vibrant, effective man.

In the beginning of time, man was looked upon as Nefer-Atum, a Lotus Man in his illuminated state. Man has since fallen from his original way and is sometimes called the "Old Dirty Bastard," so disease and violence cover the Earth.

Man needs a new day and a new way for a new Earth to rise. Over the coming days, weeks, and seasons, you will heal thyself through the wellness protocols, and they will bring man to his full bloom as he awakens the healer within. For the power to heal is within.

> "Transformation to higher ground—
> Transformation to a higher place."
>
> —KATRIEL WISE
> *The Mystic Maestro*

ACCOUNTABILITY POWER CHARGE:

Wellness Salute, Beloved Brother! You are valuable, deserving, and worthy! Continue to stand in your value as you revolutionize your rebirth! Continue to stand in your power as you metamorphize your renewal! Continue to embrace the release of all that no longer serves you! Continue to embody the courage and tenacity within you to move forward in your healing process! Continue to honor the old you who brought you to this moment! Continue to love who you are becoming, right now, right here, unconditionally! You are valuable, deserving, and worthy! You are a Wellness Warrior!

As a Wellness Warrior, you are transforming in profound and prolific ways along with your brothers within the Fraternity of Wellness. As a brotherhood, you are taking responsibility for your wellness individually as well as collectively. As you heal and set an example of optimal wellness, your brother will heal and set an example of optimal wellness. So, you are working in tandem with your brotherhood, growing and developing together. You are building! You are unifying!

Through your transformation and your renewal, you are stacking your wellness. You are training and delivering results because of your commitment to yourself and to your brotherhood. You are refining and systemizing a wellness regimen that holistically supports your mind, body, and spirit. You are celebrating your victories! You are feeling lighter and more virile!

As a Black Man, you are the most elevated man on Earth, as you are the first healer on Earth. As a Black Man, you have been seen as Nefer-Atum, a Lotus Man in his illuminated state.

Yet . . . as a Black Man, you are statistically the most traumatized from 400 years of chattel slavery. As a Black Man, you have agonized as a casualty of a stolen legacy. As a Black Man, you have endured the highest proportions of all disease, including economic starvation, emotional and psychological deprivation, and dietary malnutrition. As a Black Man, you have suffered from the highest incidences of diabetes, high blood pressure, stroke, heart disease, kidney failure, impotence, depression, and premature death.

For you, the first man of humanity, this time is yours! Rise Up! Overcome! Be counted in wellness!

The time is here to make a global shift from using power that destroys to power that builds. For power that destroys, especially in these current times, creates massive and unrelenting disease, greed, violence, and widespread destruction to nature and to humanity. This destruction is reflected and expressed through domination, suppression, oppression, and manipulation.

Power that builds is true power, yielding inner harmony,

optimal health, and balanced wealth. Ma'at is what the Ancient Nile Valley ancestors called this state of balance, truth, righteousness, and reciprocity. As you apply the teachings in this text, you will attain alignment. You will attract abundance into your life like a magnet through your powerful and reaffirming thoughts, words, actions, and deeds. You will blossom like a lotus as you continue to transform and to renew.

Through your mental, physical, emotional, social, and sexual elevation, you will shift the current conditions on Earth from toxic people, toxic land, and toxic environment to holistic people who will restore the Earth. Through your elevation and raising of your frequency, you will cause the air and water to purify and the Earth to recover in minerals and mass. Each day that you grow in wellness, you will blossom and shift from an impotent, confused, weak, unsure, ineffective man to a potent, empowered, healthy, vibrant, and effective man.

A new day and a new way are needed for a new Earth to rise. Over the coming days, weeks, and seasons, you will heal thyself through wellness protocols. You will help to bring humanity to its full bloom as you awaken the healer within you. For the mighty power to heal is within you. You are a mighty and powerful healer!

> "As above, so below, as within, so without, as the universe, so the soul . . ."
>
> —THOTH
> *Kemetic Deity*

> "The first person you have to resurrect is yourself."
>
> —RZA
> *American Musician, Rapper, Record Producer, Actor, Filmmaker, and Author*

ACCOUNTABILITY POWER CHARGE ASSIGNMENT:

PART 1: IDENTIFY DAILY PERSONAL ROADBLOCKS

- Identify and write down 3 to 5 things that are blocking your transformation daily.
- What obstacles are you encountering daily that are throwing you off your commitment to your daily wellness rituals?
- What roadblocks are stopping you from prioritizing your self-care?
- What are the inner challenges that you are facing when you are not showing up for yourself 100 percent every day?
- What are the outer challenges that you are facing when you are not showing up for yourself 100 percent every day?

PART 2: CREATING SOLUTIONS TO OVERCOME PERSONAL ROADBLOCKS

- Meditate and write down 3 to 5 solutions that you can begin to implement immediately to address the daily personal roadblocks that you identified and wrote down for Part 1 of this assignment.
- What is your remedy for overcoming your obstacles in executing your daily wellness rituals?
- What steps can you take to hold yourself accountable for executing your daily wellness rituals?
- What do you need in place to set yourself up for success in executing your daily wellness rituals?
- What specific tasks can you complete to show up for yourself 100 percent each and every day?

PART 3: ACCOUNTABILITY POWER CHARGE AFFIRMATION

- Review what you wrote for Parts 1 and 2 of this assignment, where you identified your daily personal roadblocks and your solutions to remedy those blockages.

- Create your own personal Accountability Power Charge Affirmation that will hold you accountable for achieving your optimal wellness and self-mastery.
- Write down 2 to 3 lines/sentences to affirm your action steps to overcome and to release your daily personal roadblocks.
- How can you set yourself up for success every single day in executing your daily wellness rituals?
- What do you need to remind yourself every day to feel successful in executing your daily wellness rituals?

Examples:

— I, Halleluyah Walcott, am more than the habits that I use as a crutch. I am whole. I am mighty. I create my reality every minute of every day. I am worthy of the creation of my optimal life.

— I, Zakai, affirm my discipline and dedication to stay on my wellness path every day, hour, minute, and second to achieve optimal wellness with my mind, body, and spirit.

— I, Shawn, will start my day by praising myself. I will focus on me by exercising my mind, body, and spirit to move forward in life with purpose and promise. I will limit my access to people, places, and things that will hinder my destiny.

PRACTICE:

— Take a few moments to affirm yourself daily.

— Affirm yourself in the morning when you rise and in the night before you fall into slumber.

— Both in the morning and in the night, repeat your Accountability Power Charge Affirmation to yourself

3 times: 1 time for your mind, 1 time for your body, and 1 time for your spirit.

ARIT 3: THE TRANSFORMATION MAN DAILY SPIRITUAL OBSERVANCES

ARIT POWER CENTER: SOLAR PLEXUS—LIVER, PANCREAS, AND BACK

ARIT COLOR: YELLOW

1. **THE SPIRITUAL BATH**

2. **AROMATHERAPY**

3. **YOUR ALTAR**

4. **ARIT 3 AFFIRMATION:**

   "Come forth
   . . . Make the transformation."
   —*The Papyrus of Ani*

5. **LIBATION**

6. **MAN HEAL THYSELF WELLNESS WARRIOR PRAYER**

7. **SOLAR PLEXUS EMPOWERMENT AFFIRMATION—ARIT 3:**

   May my solar plexus, the house of my kidneys, liver, pancreas, and back, function in optimal wellness. May I grow from all my experiences and come into greater awareness of my power so that I can heal myself. May I absorb, assimilate, digest, process, release, and let go completely and fully so that I may be elevated beyond excess. May I not be immersed in toxicity due to my challenging life experiences. May I receive a clear understanding of what I create so that I may receive and grow abundantly throughout my life in purpose, passion, and prosperity.

8. **CHANT (HESI)**

9. **FIRE BREATHS**

10. **HEALING STONE MEDITATION AND VISUALIZATION**

11. **HERBAL TONICS**

12. **WELLNESS WARRIOR JOURNAL WRITING**

13. **AFFIRMATION CONFIRMATION**

14. **PRAYER OF FORGIVENESS**

15. **PROBLEM-SOLVER AFFIRMATIONS**

16. **EXERCISE: COMPLETE YOUR WORKOUT FROM THE MAN HEAL THYSELF 12-WEEK WORKOUT PLAN**

ARIT 4: THE LOVER MAN OF HARMONY

> "I am pure of heart within a pure body.
> I exist in my heart. May my heart not be taken from me.
> Let it not be wounded . . . I know my heart.
> I have gained power over my heart."
>
> —THE PAPYRUS OF ANI

LOVING OURSELVES; LOVING YOU

Just when I thought I was finished writing this book, *Man, Heal Thyself*, I attended a women's creative/political event. In the late evening after a very long day, I took a cab from Brooklyn to Harlem—I had been invited by a sister-friend, and I had to get there to show my support for the women presenting the event. I jumped out of the cab and hurried through a steady rain into a crowded, dimly lit room. Black women and women of all races and political orientations, wounded women, were in attendance in the room and expressing their feelings.

I was familiar with this room; I have been in rooms like this most of my life. It was my mother's kitchen, my girlfriend's living room, my auntie's dining room. In those rooms, women talk about you: the men we used to love; the one we love now; the men we want to love; the men we are done loving. Sometimes it's so deep that we try to talk the love away just to stop the pain of loving. In the room this rainy Friday night, there was a circle of women and a few men who cared to be there. Upon entering, I paused; I could feel what was there and what was to come. It was on the walls and in the air. I almost could not breathe as I was pulled into the heart of the room where women were talking out loud with hard, beating breaths—about you. Woman after woman took center stage and "ripped off her skin" in front of herself and her sisters and the men who had cared to be there and were listening. Poetically, courageously, the women revealed their hidden rage. Each one shouted, screamed, wept, moaned, and hollered to release the pain she had kept silenced for too long. Her sisters and the men who had cared to be there watched on.

Some of these women were running to men in the hopes that this time it would be different from the last time. Others were running from lovers, husbands, friends, partners—running for their lives. They had become afraid of themselves in the state of unresolved fear that they saw reflected on your face. Untreated fear had converted into rage . . . and the rage had converted into war. The Gender War. Man against woman and woman against man; the Gender War is swords pressed into each other until we bleed. It is women thrusting angry faces; it is deep-seated, heart-bursting anger. It is generations of pain. In the room, artists, poets, dancers expressed the back-breaking madness of the Gender War with pulsating sounds, body-beating dance movements, and words that thundered like stomping feet and bass drums. They hit the floor with bare-fisted protests against the ongoing pain of unhealthy unions. They held their limbs in deformed positions to express "Loving him hurts so bad, I'm feeling sad and broken." Their songs and dances said, "Man/Woman, loving is natural, but we have been so overexposed to the unnatural that we would rather maim and kill with looks and attitudes and words than be in pain in the name of love."

We women want to love you real good, but we have been literally and figuratively beaten and raped in the name of politics, social justice, and economics—and even in the name of love. Bad lovin' has wounded our hearts, attacked our wombs, and made us . . . mad. "That's enough!" the women were saying in their poems and dances that night.

Man, Heal Thyself. Listen to the women as they tell, we tell what is hurting us. You can't heal you if you can't hear us, if you don't even listen to us. I am you, and you are me. We are the reflection of each other.

What I create is equally your creation. Such are the natural laws of Gender Peace.

So, just when I thought I was finished writing this book, *Man, Heal Thyself*, I went to a women's event. They were in a room talking about themselves and about you. And because I am the Velvet Sword, and because this book is about men healing themselves, I had to write this article and tell you what we women are saying and thinking and feeling about loving ourselves while loving you . . .

—*Queen Afua*

"There's a mystic seed that grows through a space
that no one knows in the heart of man.
It nourishes the soul if allowed to unfold in the heart of man."

—LADY PREMA

Crystal Sage Woman

OPENING THE WAY:

The Lover Man represents unconditional love. He has unconditional love for himself and for others. He is deeply connected to himself and deeply bonded with others. His love flows from within first, so that love can easily flow from him. He emits a harmonious and joyous exchange of energy with all that is around him. His open and brave heart is filled with love, compassion, forgiveness, mercy, empathy, and acceptance. The Lover Man has the capacity to truly love as he leads from his heart, speaks from his heart, listens from his heart, and acts from his heart.

The Lover Man is filled with the pure spirit of the Most High. He easily downloads divine love from above to spread love throughout. The Lover Man can bring wholeness through integration and unification between earthly and spiritual aspirations. He recognizes that he is interconnected to an intricate web of relationships expanding throughout life and the universe. The Lover Man is in alignment with the sacred and essential truth that flows through all of life and links everything together.

The Lover Man understands the importance of reciprocity and balance when it comes to matters of the heart. He lives a heart-centered life where love is both given and received. This balance purifies his personal needs and desires, allowing him to open his heart and to embrace vulnerability for deeper connection with others.

The Lover Man heals the broken hearts of wounded souls who are seeking to be whole. He mends the damaged spirits requiring renewal. The Lover Man carries with him a fiery heart that dissolves the rage of fibroid tumors growing within the wombs of the women he loves.

The Lover Man honors and respects, restores and rejuvenates. He is trustworthy and transparent; he says what he means and means what he says. He cherishes and appreciates others, carefully safeguarding their hearts.

The Lover Man creates a safe haven within his body for vulnerability to exist with his beloved. He nourishes his beloved mentally, emotionally, spiritually, and sexually. His love is self-generating like the Sun. The Lover Man fills the world with music, song, poetry, and dance with every thought, word, action, and deed. He pours love into the air, mystically creating profound balance, peace, harmony, truth, and order.

The Lover Man of Harmony dwells in the Green Heart Center that houses the nervous system, bloodstream, and heart. Among African Americans, 31.7 percent have hypertension. Among Hispanics or Latinos, 20.6 percent have hypertension. Among African Americans, 10.2 percent have heart disease (HD), 6.0 percent have chronic heart disease (CHD). Among Hispanics or Latinos, 8.8 percent have a coronary heart defect (CHD).

HEART-CENTERED:

Wellness Salute, Dear Brother! We—you, me, and our brotherhood—are working together. We are the seekers of becoming better men. We are unifying, strengthening, and establishing ourselves as a community of men who are on the frontlines of wellness. We are choosing to pour into ourselves daily. We are choosing to hold ourselves accountable. We are choosing to live a holistic plant-based lifestyle. We are choosing to use herbs and nature's cures to heal and to remove disease from our body temples. We are choosing to shatter the walls and layers that we have built around our hearts. We are choosing to forgive ourselves for being human. We are choosing to forgive others for being human just like us. We are choosing to release all that no longer serves us. We are choosing to let go of everything that is holding us back from standing in our true power. We are choosing to surrender. We are choosing to be alpha men.

We, as men, have a responsibility to learn how to be open with our hearts. We, as men, have a responsibility to learn how to speak from our hearts more effectively. We, as men, have a responsibility to tell our stories, our truths from our hearts to the women and men in our lives without fear, shame, and guilt. We, as men, have a responsibility to be vulnerable by really saying what we mean and really meaning what we say. We, as men, have a responsibility to express our hearts through our actions of love. We, as men, have a responsibility to love responsibly and completely with our full and whole hearts.

Beloved Brother, the truth is that we are the key to shifting our relationships. We must recognize that self-love is essential to this shift. We must love ourselves unconditionally and with complete acceptance. We must forgive the men we were yesterday and embrace who we are right now. We want balance, peace, harmony, truth, and order within our households, with our mates, with our families, with our friends. As men, we are doers, mighty and powerful problem-solvers. So, to achieve Ma'at, we must be in alignment with both the divine feminine and divine masculine within each of us. We must tap into our compassion and empathy. We must be fearless in entering the world of our emotions and feelings. We must be courageous in leading our words and actions from our open and brave hearts.

As men, standing in our power means to speak our truths candidly and courageously from our hearts. Being brave and fearless with sharing our emotions and feelings to the women and men in our lives is strength, not weakness. Acknowledging and expressing our stories to others increases our power, value, and fortitude.

To truly heal, we must break the cycle. We must break the chains. We must end the Gender War. We must stop hurting and pushing away our women because of our fears and our egos. We are stronger and better than that. We are Wellness Warriors!

We are the only ones who can stop the pain that our women are carrying around because of the men in their lives. We must listen to the women as they tell us what is hurting them. We must open our hearts to hear their painful truths. We must be resilient in showing our empathy and our compassion, even though our women's words may be hard to digest. We have an opportunity to build, to grow, and to heal.

In return, Beloved Brother, we have an opportunity to share the pain that we are carrying around because of the women in our lives. We must tell the women what is hurting us. We must open our hearts to speak our painful truths. We must be resilient in showing ourselves empathy and compassion even though our words may be hard to communicate. We have an opportunity to build, to grow, and to heal.

I am you. You are me. We are them. They are us. We are each the reflection of the other. What I create is equally your creation. What you create is equally my creation. What we create is equally their creation. What they create is equally our creation.

Love and Light. Mer and Ra.

HEART-CENTERED ASSIGNMENT:

PRAYER OF FORGIVENESS REVISIT

- Review the Prayer of Forgiveness you wrote at the beginning of Arit 1: The Family Man of Unity and Wealth.
- Revise your Prayer of Forgiveness. Go deeper into your healing. Allow yourself to feel and to acknowledge what you need to forgive within yourself so your heart opens and shines brightly.
- Hold yourself accountable while releasing self-judgment and self-criticism.

PART 2: IDENTIFYING CHALLENGES IN OUR RELATIONSHIPS WITH WOMEN

- Identify and write down 3 to 5 of the biggest challenges that you have encountered in your relationships with women.
  - — What are challenges that men and women experience when interacting with each other?
  - — What do both men and women need to do to interact with each other in a more balanced and harmonious way?
  - — What obstacles do you face in your relationships with the women in your life?
  - — What is at the root of your disharmony with the women in your life?

PART 3: DEFINING LOVE

- Identify and write down 3 to 5 definitions of love.
  - — What does love mean to you?
  - — What do you need to feel loved?
  - — What do you need to do for others to feel and to experience your love?

— How do you see love?
— How do you want to be loved?
— How do you want to love?

PART 4: DEFINING EXPECTATIONS IN TERMS OF LOVE AND ROMANCE

- Review what you wrote for Parts 1, 2, and 3 of this assignment, where you revised your Prayer of Forgiveness, identified challenges in your relationships with the women in your life, and defined what love means to you.
- Identify and write down 3 to 5 expectations you have in a sacred union.
  — What do you expect from yourself as a life partner?
  — What do you expect from your beloved as a life partner?
  — What are the qualities you expect in a sacred union for balance, peace, harmony, truth, and order to exist?
  — What is love for you in a sacred union?
  — What do you ultimately want when it comes to matters of love and romance?

The true Lover Man is not a womanizer, a rolling stone, or a heartbreaker. The Lover Man is filled with the pure spirit of the Most High. He has a huge heart filled with love, mercy, compassion, and forgiveness.

The Lover Man heals the broken hearts of wounded souls. A Lover Man honors and respects, restores not damages, and is trustworthy rather than dishonest. A Lover Man is not a double talker; he says what he means and means what he says. You can trust him with your heart.

The Lover Man fills the world with music, poetry, song, and dance with every thought, word, and deed. He pours love into the air. In the body of the Lover Man there exists a safe haven—a place in him that you can trust to be honest. The

Lover Man will nourish you mentally, emotionally, spiritually, and sexually. Even when at his worst state, one cannot take away from the Lover Man because his love is self-generating like the Sun.

The Lover Man carries within him a fiery heart that dissolves the rage of a fibroid tumor, a wounded heart that is seeking to be whole, or a broken spirit that needs mending. The touch of the Lover Man makes the coldest soul warm again. The Lover Man is his own healer, and he can heal himself, leaving him free of heart disease and strokes. A Lover Man of Soul Beauty will mystically bring you into a harmony profound.

ARIT 4: THE LOVER MAN DAILY SPIRITUAL OBSERVANCES

ARIT POWER CENTER: HEART, CIRCULATORY SYSTEM, AND LUNGS
ARIT COLOR: GREEN

1. **THE SPIRITUAL BATH**

2. **AROMATHERAPY**

3. **YOUR ALTAR**

4. **ARIT 4 AFFIRMATION:**

   "I am pure of heart within a pure body.
   I exist in my heart.
   May my heart not be taken from me. Let it not be wounded . . . I know my heart.
   I have gained power over my heart."

   —THE PAPYRUS OF ANI

5. **LIBATION**

6. **MAN HEAL THYSELF WELLNESS WARRIOR PRAYER**

7. **HEART/THYMUS EMPOWERMENT AFFIRMATION—ARIT 4:**
May my heart center that houses my bloodstream, nervous system, circulatory system, lungs, and back function in optimal wellness. May my heart be not imbalanced, wounded, and heavy. May my heart be in Ma'at (balanced, harmonious, forgiving). With each experience, may I breathe deep and full breaths in all that I do. May all my relations be renewed through my healthy heart. May I be released from heart attacks and heart murmurs. May healthy thoughts travel into my heart and help me maintain a huge heart of mercy and compassion for myself and all my relationships.

8. **CHANT (HESI)**

9. **FIRE BREATHS**

10. **HEALING STONE MEDITATION AND VISUALIZATION**

11. **HERBAL TONICS**

12. **WELLNESS WARRIOR JOURNAL WRITING**

13. **AFFIRMATION CONFIRMATION**

14. **PRAYER OF FORGIVENESS**

15. **PROBLEM-SOLVER AFFIRMATIONS**

16. **VALUE AND POWER AFFIRMATIONS**

17. **ACCOUNTABILITY POWER CHARGE AFFIRMATION CONFIRMATION**

18. **LOVE AFFIRMATIONS**

19. **EXERCISE: COMPLETE YOUR WORKOUT FROM THE MAN HEAL THYSELF 12-WEEK WORKOUT PLAN**

ARIT 5: THE COMMUNICATION MAN OF CONNECTIVITY AND CREATIVITY

> "I speak that I wish to become strong and I come into existence as I speak.
> I have commanded my seat.
> I rule it by my mouth."
>
> —THE PAPYRUS OF ANI

OPENING THE WAY:

The Communication Man authentically expresses his truth through his words, embracing his originality. He lives a life of personal integrity with a strong sense of honor. He communicates his thoughts, feelings, and intentions clearly, effectively, and accurately. He says what he means and means what he says. He affirms himself daily, breathing words of power, strength, and confidence into his mind, body, and spirit.

The Communication Man is aligned with himself and the Most High. He tunes in and listens to the guidance of his Highest Self. He knows his inner truth. He communicates and lives his truth daily.

The Communication Man stands in his power with an open heart. He speaks with intention. He communicates with transparency and honesty. He advocates for himself and his beliefs. He establishes boundaries, saying no when needed. The Communication Man is balanced in truth and authenticity.

The Communication Man is an active listener. He listens deeply to others, gifting the experience of being heard. He is focused, present, and patient. He listens for connection. He listens to understand. He listens to learn. He listens to gather information. He listens with curiosity. He listens with pleasure. He listens with compassion. The Communication Man listens without judgment. He listens with acceptance and openness.

The Communication Man speaks words of encouragement. His words inspire others to live life to the fullest. His words are spoken with strength and conviction, with love and understanding. His words are manifestations of his soul.

The Communication Man speaks words as medicine. His words help others to remove themselves from harm's way. His words raise others from the depths of the Earth. His words inspire others to transcend apparent limitations.

The Communication Man can shape and reshape life, people, environments, places, and things with his words. He can enter a body temple and speak wellness into a sick soul. The Communication Man eases pain with his healing words. He shifts minds and clears mad thoughts through his positive and affirmative words. He opens the way to those who have lost direction and creates new pathways using his charge-conscious words.

The Communication Man dwells in the throat center, which houses the lungs and throat. African American men in particular are at risk; they are 37 percent more likely to develop lung cancer than white men. African American men have the highest incidence of throat cancer (approximately 12 percent).

OUR WORDS, OUR POWER:

Wellness Salute, King! We—you, me, and our brotherhood—are collectively working together to shed the energies that no longer serve us. We are creating pathways to activate and to actualize each of the Arit, energy centers. We are calibrating to take action and to forge ahead. We are clearing the way and saying goodbye to the clutter. We are releasing the old, inadequate, and unproductive aspects of who we are through our shared energies of empowerment. We are falling in love with ourselves more and more as we surrender to the Most High and as we maintain our commitment to our self-masteries. We are elevating and aligning. We are building. We are electrifying ourselves, our brotherhood, our relationships, and our communities.

As Wellness Warriors, we are assembled like the mighty avengers of our ancestors committed to being examples in this revolution of absolute change and holistic polarity on this planet. We have been chosen by our ancestors to break the chains. In doing so, we must recognize that as men in Western society, we are trained daily to make personal sacrifices. We are taught to place our true value below our true potential. We are expected to make the ultimate sacrifice—to place the value of people, places, and things far above ourselves. This lack of value and lack of knowing ourselves makes us internally self-destruct. Consequently, we lash out. We hurt ourselves. We hurt our loved ones. We hurt our communities. Our self-destruction, our self-sabotage, our self-slaughter stop now!

We must get to a point where we win without hesitation. We are being hunted globally. We are being destroyed by health disparities, the law, opposing tribes, anything and anyone who wants to prevent us from realizing who we really are. We are being stopped from standing in our mighty power. We say no more! We say no more to being the prey!

Instead of continuing our lineages of pain and hurt, my Dear Brother, speak your mighty power onto yourself. Speak the collective power of all our mightiness onto all of us. We are the first value. Everything first starts with us. We must remember and internalize our sacredness and worthiness. We must claim ourselves! We must continue to affirm ourselves! Our words are our power!

We are birthing the new world from the consciousness of our minds. Every man, no matter race or creed, must deem himself valuable and deserving. We must deploy this value and power onto all our relations and the world. We must shine in our brilliance through our immortality. We must prioritize our self-care. We must embrace self-love.

As we pour into ourselves, our hearts are opening to experience the greatest emotions and feelings of love that we will ever know. We are becoming more expansive. We are ready to receive. We are doing this work!

We are healing ourselves! We are winning! We are experiencing the jewels of the Most High filtering through us. We are showering ourselves with inspiration and motivation. We are thriving as men, as kings, as brothers! We recognize what being a man is and what being a man entails. We are standing in our power. We are rising boldly in our A-tone as alpha men.

We have everything we will ever need seeded within us to create the world we want and we desire. We are aligning with being true to our blessed divine nature. We are rejuvenated, reenergized, and renewed. We are abundant. Our words are the conduit for which we, alpha men, affirm our power onto ourselves and onto the world. Our words are our truths. Our words are our bonds. Our words are our spells. We speak our power into existence through our words. We speak life into ourselves and each other through our words. We speak our truth and express our divinity through our words. Our words are potent and powerful.

> "There is not a path to wellness; wellness is the path."
>
> —DEDRIC AVERY
>
> *Man Heal Thyself Wellness Warrior,*
> *Inaugural Class, Spring 2020*

OUR WORDS, OUR POWER ASSIGNMENT:

PART 1: IDENTIFY COMMUNICATION BLOCKAGES

- Identify and write down 5 blockages that you have around communication in your life.
  - What is holding you back from fully communicating yourself to others?
  - What obstacles do you encounter when you share information with others?
  - What challenges do you experience when you receive information from others?
  - What keeps you from being transparent in your communication?
  - What prevents you from communicating clearly, concisely, and effectively?
  - What traumas have you experienced around your words, your voice, and your power?

PART 2: CREATE ACTION STEPS TO RESTORE YOUR COMMUNICATION

- Meditate and write down 5 solutions that you can begin to implement immediately to restore your communication.
  - What is your remedy for overcoming your obstacles in executing better communication?
  - What action steps can you take to hold yourself accountable for executing better communication?
  - What do you need in place to set yourself up for success in executing better communication?
  - What qualities of excellent communication do you need to embrace to be a better communicator?

PART 3: SEND ENERGY TO YOUR THROAT

- Send energy to your throat.
- Place the back of your hands on your throat and exhale.
- Breath intentional life into your throat and your body.

ARIT 5: THE COMMUNICATION MAN DAILY SPIRITUAL OBSERVANCES

ARIT POWER CENTER: THROAT, THYROID, SHOULDERS, AND NECK

ARIT COLOR: BLUE

1. **THE SPIRITUAL BATH**

2. **AROMATHERAPY**

3. **YOUR ALTAR**

4. **ARIT 5 AFFIRMATION:**

   "I speak that I wish to become strong, and I come into existence as I speak.
   I have commanded my seat.
   I rule it by my mouth."

   —THE PAPYRUS OF ANI

5. **LIBATION**

6. **MAN HEAL THYSELF WELLNESS WARRIOR PRAYER**

7. **EMPOWERMENT AND DETOXIFICATION AFFIRMATION—ARIT 5:**
   May my thyroid center, which houses my throat, function in optimal wellness. May I speak myself into wholeness from limb to limb. I now speak words of power, words of strength, words of renewal, words to uplift every body member. May my body, mind, and spirit respond with assurance. For my mind and heart

are connected to my words and my body is connected to my entire anatomy. My body and my words are one. I send messages of wellness and aliveness to each muscle, nerve, bone, and joint. My body honors the words from my mouth. I have the power within me to speak through my words a new relationship, a new life, a new world.

8. **CHANT (HESI)**
9. **FIRE BREATHS**
10. **HEALING STONE MEDITATION AND VISUALIZATION**
11. **HERBAL TONICS**
12. **WELLNESS WARRIOR JOURNAL WRITING**
13. **AFFIRMATION CONFIRMATION**
14. **PRAYER OF FORGIVENESS**
15. **PROBLEM-SOLVER AFFIRMATIONS**
16. **VALUE AND POWER AFFIRMATIONS**
17. **ACCOUNTABILITY POWER CHARGE AFFIRMATION CONFIRMATION**
18. **LOVE AFFIRMATIONS**
19. **COMMUNICATION AFFIRMATIONS**
20. **EXERCISE: COMPLETE YOUR WORKOUT FROM THE MAN HEAL THYSELF 12-WEEK WORKOUT PLAN**

ARIT 6: THE INTUITIVE MAN OF CLEAR VISION

"Open my eyes I've been blind.
I live in the utchat.
I live by its strength.
My intuition is powerful."

—THE PAPYRUS OF ANI

OPENING THE WAY:

The Intuitive Man is a fully awakened and activated man of consciousness. His left brain and his right brain function in synchronicity. His creativity and synthetic thinking are balanced and unified with his logical and analytical thinking. He is a visionary who transcends time, having the ability to connect with both the inner and outer worlds of spirit and self. His thinking is clear, as he receives spiritual messages and self-reflective downloads.

The Intuitive Man navigates a journey within, inwardly exploring himself and clearing the way to receive as he pours into himself. He connects to the spirit deepest inside of himself, guiding him to acquire deeper truths that transcend the mind and surpass words.

The Intuitive Man is mighty and powerful. He is open to intuitive sensibilities and inner perceptions. He is enhanced by his inner guidance. He possesses both the seat of wisdom and the seat of conscience. The Intuitive Man has a lucid knowingness of the heart and the soul. He can see, hear, and interpret the words from silent thoughts. He can decipher the past and look clearly into the future. The Intuitive Man trusts himself to be a knower.

The Intuitive Man lives in the spirit and by the spirit. He meditates to find stillness in order to listen to the Most High and to meet his true self, the one who has been whispering words of greatness and empowerment to him. He accesses his inner wisdom easily, as he has built a relationship trusting the voice within him.

The Intuitive Man is in alignment with his inner voice, which is the expression of his most inspired and ingenious self. He hears and listens to the voice of his highest soul self. The Intuitive Man is guided to a life of eminence through his inner voice. His inner voice carries him through his life's journey. His genius and creativity emerge from a heart filled with gratitude, for he celebrates his Godhead and honors the unconditional love he has for the Most High.

The Intuitive Man feeds his conscious and subconscious mind with inversion exercises, meditations, daily prayers, and green plant foods that develop his intuitive gifts and strengthen his psychic knowledge.

The Intuitive Man is one who is a seer and who can hear the words from your silent thoughts and interpret them. One who can decipher your past and look clearly into your future. The Intuitive Man trusts himself to be a knower. The Intuitive Man lives in the spirit and by the spirit. The Intuitive Man is connected to his inner voice, and that voice carries him through his life's journey.

The Intuitive Man dwells in the indigo pineal energy center that houses the mouth, eyes, and face. Glaucoma is the most common cause of blindness among people of African descent. They often develop glaucoma early in life, and they tend to have a more aggressive form of the disease.

PERSPICUITY:

Wellness Salute, Almighty! We—you, me, and our brotherhood—have created a formation that is functioning synchronistically to achieve our individual and collective self-mastery. Our formation will save our lives. Every day is a challenge to heal ourselves. We are staying bonded as a result. We are holding ourselves and each other accountable to executing our daily wellness protocols. We are committed to our commitments even more passionately now. We are our brothers' keepers. We are feeding each other. We are supporting each other. We are speaking life into ourselves and into each other. When we come together as men, as brothers, as kings, as Godheads, we are charging and energizing each other, our families, and our planet. We are connecting! We are elevating!

From sperm to egg, we have been deployed to this glorious

planet, Earth. We have been given the audacious opportunity to contribute to the divine creation story. Our daily wellness protocols are designed to cultivate self-mastery. With our discipline, we are the best versions of ourselves. When we are at our finest, we are embodying the original intent of our creation orders. Let's maximize our time, great brother. Let's continue to grow and to develop in the highest vibrations of love and light until we transform out of our physical powerhouses back into our star bodies. In doing so, we are setting our daily intentions and activating ourselves first and foremost. We want to be of greater service to ourselves and the Most High so that we can serve the ones we love as well as the world.

As we navigate our healing and transformations, we are experiencing a variety of breakthroughs. We are each coming into being. As we build and evolve, we are standing strong and embracing our power with graciousness, gratitude, and contentment. We are divorcing ourselves from expectations outside of ourselves. We are silencing the internal critics standing on our shoulders who are self-sabotaging our progress and discipline. We are recognizing the responsibility we have to ourselves to transmute all negative energies that are obstacles for our healing. When we transmute the low vibrations, we are diving deeper into Spirit for clarity. We are building our muscles—our mind, body, and spirit muscles. We are strengthening our life force and energetic space. We are changing the chemistry of perception.

As we are claiming who we are as men, we are owning ourselves. We are reestablishing our own personal ministries. We are enshrining ourselves as our own personal Godheads. We are loving ourselves at the highest level. We are centered and balanced. We are embracing every aspect of who we are, both our righteousness and our sins. We are practicing forgiveness. We are trusting our intuition and our instincts. We are releasing all that no longer serves us. We are eliminating our burdens to be lighter. We are clearing the path for our antennas, our spiritual receptors, to be open to receive our spiritual visions, our spiritual downloads, our spiritual messages from the Most High.

As men, we are being watched and observed. As Wellness Warriors, we are being watched and observed. We have a responsibility to ourselves and to each other to recognize and acknowledge that we are on a stage. Let this sink in. Marinate in the responsibility and accountability of what this stage means, beloved brother. We have an opportunity and an obligation to perform at our highest and mightiest. In doing so, we are remembering who we are. We are resilient, powerful men. We are erect in our apexes. We are manifesting and exhibiting the qualities and characteristics of what it means to be alpha men.

"Allow me to re-introduce myself."

—JAY-Z

American Rapper, Songwriter, Record Executive, Businessman, and Record Producer

PERSPICUITY ASSIGNMENT:

PART 1: IDENTIFY CLEAR VISION BLOCKAGES

- Identify and write down 3 blockages that have been obstructing your vision and preventing you from clearly seeing your true self.
  - What in me has been hindering me from seeing clearly?
  - What in me has been limiting me from really accessing what I need to see clearly?
  - What in me has been preventing me from being centered and quiet in order to receive?
  - What in me has been blocking me from being present?
  - What in me has been inhibiting me from hearing the answers internally?
  - What is causing my brain fog?
  - Why is it challenging to meditate and to visualize what I want and seek for myself?
  - Why do I look outside myself for answers when the answers are in me?

PART 2: INNER VOICE POWER CHARGE AFFIRMATION

- Review what you wrote for Part 1 of this assignment, where you identified your clear vision blockages.
- Create your own personal Inner Voice Power Charge Affirmation that will support complete access to your spiritual visions, your spiritual downloads, your spiritual messages.
- Write down 3 to 5 lines/sentences to affirm your action steps that embrace your powerful intuition, your mighty inner voice, your magnificent Godhead.
  - How will you affirm your strength and power to claim your self-empowerment?
  - What do you need to do to remember your strength and power?

— How will you access your spiritual visions, your spiritual downloads, your spiritual messages?

Examples:

— I, Halleluyah Walcott, will recognize my utchat and respect the message enough to follow. I will shave away all indulgences that will not put me on the path to my vision. I will love myself enough to shift my inaction to action. I will direct my energy to the purpose of vision. I am a man of action. I slumber no more.

— I, Adelson, will obey my instinct. I will trust myself the same way I trust those who I hold sacred. I will refuse to dim my light and replace it with darkness. I will set my intentions directly on my highest form. I will love unconditionally inwardly as I do outwardly. I will treat me like me means the most to me. I will see me as I see my God.

— I, Enen Kes Maa, will open my eyes to the glory of myself. I will kick up my meditations and chantings to listen to the mantra of Heru the King. Heru is the will and the utchat in the center of my forehead. I will eat and drink specific foods and herbs that feed my utchat. I will continue to recognize and to get rid of all my garbage that is blocking my vision.

PRACTICE:

— Take a few moments to affirm yourself daily.

— Affirm yourself in the morning when you rise and in the night before you fall into slumber.

— Both in the morning and in the night, repeat your Inner Voice Power Charge Affirmation to yourself 3 times: 1 time for your mind, 1 time for your body, and 1 time for your spirit.

ARIT 6: THE INTUITIVE MAN DAILY SPIRITUAL OBSERVANCES

ARIT POWER CENTER: PINEAL GLAND, EYES, FACE, AND MOUTH

ARIT COLOR: INDIGO

1. **THE SPIRITUAL BATH**

2. **AROMATHERAPY**

3. **YOUR ALTAR**

4. **ARIT 6 AFFIRMATION:**

   "Open my eyes
   I've been blind.
   I live in the Utchat [my high mind] I live by its strength.
   My intuition powerful."
   —*The Papyrus of Ani*

5. **LIBATION**

6. **MAN HEAL THYSELF WELLNESS WARRIOR PRAYER**

7. **PINEAL INTUITIVE EMPOWERMENT AFFIRMATION—ARIT 6:**

   May my pineal center, which houses my intuition, face, eyes, and mouth, function in optimal wellness. May I see and speak myself into wholeness from limb to limb. May I become a clear messenger of truth. May I receive guidance and protection as I connect to my inner voice. The voice that teaches me moment by moment how to live life in complete oneness with my purpose. May I listen, trust, act, and protect my inner vision so that I may become the greatness that I was born to be. May the serenity in my eyes, the youthful expression on my face, and the peaceful words from my mouth reflect the oneness in my mind. I am a seer of clear vision.

8. **CHANT (HESI)**

9. **FIRE BREATHS**

10. **HEALING STONE MEDITATION AND VISUALIZATION**

11. **HERBAL TONICS**

12. **WELLNESS WARRIOR JOURNAL WRITING**

13. **AFFIRMATION CONFIRMATION**

14. **PRAYER OF FORGIVENESS**

15. **PROBLEM-SOLVER AFFIRMATIONS**

16. **VALUE AND POWER AFFIRMATIONS**

17. **ACCOUNTABILITY POWER CHARGE AFFIRMATION CONFIRMATION**

18. **LOVE AFFIRMATIONS**

19. **COMMUNICATION AFFIRMATIONS**

20. **RESPONSIBILITY AFFIRMATIONS**

21. **EMPOWERMENT AFFIRMATIONS**

22. **INNER VOICE POWER CHARGE AFFIRMATION**

23. **EXERCISE: COMPLETE YOUR WORKOUT FROM THE MAN HEAL THYSELF 12-WEEK WORKOUT PLAN**

ARIT 7: THE UNIVERSAL HUMANITARIAN MAN

"Emancipate yourself from mental slavery.
None but ourselves can free our minds."

—BOB MARLEY (ROBERT NESTA MARLEY)
Jamaican Singer, Songwriter, Musician,
Pioneer of Reggae

OPENING THE WAY:

The Universal Humanitarian Man is supernatural, transcendental, and enlightened. He embraces the limitless possibilities beyond the material universe. He stands in his power, eclipsing the mundane and releasing his ego. He is exceptional. The Universal Humanitarian Man is aligned, awakened, and activated. He is connected to the cosmos and to the Most High.

The Universal Humanitarian Man lives in an eternal state of unity. He perceives the world through an altruistic vision of omnipresent connection. He experiences a magical wholeness with all that he encounters, as he navigates through life. He feels unified with everyone and everything. He is in tune with nature and with the universe, always noticing the subtleties of spiritual synchronicities and mystical messages. He welcomes the interconnectedness of creation.

The Universal Humanitarian Man is an example of reciprocity. He is both a giver and receiver of life force, living in balance to merge with the collective pool of consciousness while maintaining his individuality. His energy flows freely, nourishing his mind, body, and spirit. He pours into himself as he manifests his vision of harmony for planet Earth. The Universal Humanitarian Man innerstands, understands, and overstands that he is accountable for what he creates and for what he produces. Consequently, he speaks, thinks, and acts with love, wisdom, compassion, and empathy.

The Universal Humanitarian Man, who is created from the elements (air, fire, water, and earth) and who is birthed from the sun, stars, and moon, exists in a state of optimal wellness where his potent energy flows clockwise. He is free of disease, free of toxicity, free of pain, free of suffering, and free of lack. The Universal Humanitarian Man is abundant, empowered, liberated, and healthy.

The Universal Humanitarian Man is devoted to the Divine Creator, expressing his gratitude and unconditional love for all the blessings and lessons that have shaped who he is. Because of his devotion, gratitude, and unconditional love, the Universal Humanitarian Man receives optimal guidance and preeminent knowledge from the Divine Creator. As a result, he is in alignment with supreme consciousness.

The Universal Humanitarian Man is familiar with rebirth and transformation. He easily sheds his old skin to become new. He experiences euphoric epiphanies and rapturous revelations.

BETTER THAN, MORE THAN:

Wellness Salute, Victorious! We—you, me, and our brotherhood—have an obligation to be the shining lights within the darkness and chaos. We have been called to be better than, more than. We are each more than just a Black man. We are each more than just a man. We are each so much more than just the color of our skin. We are each so much more than just our gender. We are each so much more than just where we live. We are all just human, existing on one planet, Mother Earth.

We have all been born into war, every last one of us. Every soul on this planet. Everyone. We have all been born into conflict, hostility, struggle, strife, aggression, destruction. In the happy times, in the chaos, we are all born into war, born into survival. Yet, how we choose to deploy every day into the light will determine how we navigate the discord. We must stand in our Godhead. We must be on our guard. For we are Gods on guard.

Our planet, as well as our communities, is in a state of turmoil. Stop making excuses! We were born with a foot on our necks. We have always been fighting for our breath. While we are alive, we are breathing and fighting for our survival! Those who cannot breathe are our ancestors. We must honor and celebrate our ancestors. We must allow ourselves to receive the inspiring messages that our ancestors are breathing into us every day. Many of them sacrificed themselves for us to be here today. So, as long as we can breathe and fight, we are able to see and to channel. We can plan, plot, and strategize. We can stand our ground, planting our seeds and watching them grow abundantly. As long as we are breathing and fighting, we are activating our wills and clarifying our visions. We are manifesting and transforming ourselves and our planet. For we are the chosen ones.

Make no mistake. There is nowhere to run and nowhere to hide in the cosmology. Even Heaven on Earth must be defended and fought for. Utopia is not going to be just given. Everything we need, we must work for. Everything we work for, we must protect. Whether the chaos is internal, external, or both, we must have a plan of action, a vision.

As we depart our homes and voyage into the world, we must protect ourselves in order to survive and to return home. For protection, my beloved brother, do a mind, body, and spirit check. We must leave our homes in harmony. No matter what. As soon as we leave our homes, our sanctuaries, we are subject to attacks and to uncertainties that affect our minds, bodies, and spirits. The energy we signal out into the world will return to us, so be mindful. It is essential to activate our aura fields, to make peace, and to center ourselves every day when we leave our homes. Upon returning home, we must do an energetic spiritual cleanse to avoid the transfer of outside energies into our home spaces. Execute a gratitude meditation, giving thanks for returning home safe and sound. Beloved brother, change the water on your altar, light a candle, and recite your affirmation confirmations to yourself and in celebration of your ancestors and your protective spirit guardians.

We must be the antithesis to the chaos. To create the world that we envision, we have a responsibility to be the best version of ourselves for the globe. In doing so, we are all accountable for our own minds and our own hearts. We have the power to raise ourselves up to the highest peaks where our minds are free and our hearts are light. Reaching that pinnacle of mental freedom with a light heart is what our ultimate goal is as a human. As we achieve the limitless possibilities of what we are each capable of mentally, physically, and spiritually with the liberation of our minds and our hearts, all the issues, conflicts, darkness, and chaos begin to disappear. Yet the work, our work, our Wellness Warrior spirit continues to be the driving force for our journeys to self-mastery. We are disciplined. We are diligent. We are tenacious.

As we commit even deeper to our commitment to each other and to our wellness, we learn to embrace discomfort and to find power within. We discover that discomfort is what motivates and mobilizes us into action. Without discomfort, we become complacent and accepting of the darkness and chaos where we continue to create levels of separation and differences. Instead, we use discomfort to grow and to develop, to build unity, harmony, and balance.

As Wellness Warriors, we have been deployed to lead the march of pushing forward to heal and evolve. Our commitment to our commitment will continue to expand as we dive deeper into our healing and our wellness. We are alphas! We are standing empowered in our alpha mindset, honoring our Godhead. Who we are and what we think set the example. We have the power to set the tone.

"Plan, plot, strategize, but bomb first."

—TUPAC AMARU SHAKUR (2PAC)

American Rapper, Songwriter, and Actor

BETTER THAN, MORE THAN ASSIGNMENT:

PART 1: GLOBAL WELLNESS VISION FOR HUMANITY

- What is your vision for the global wellness of humanity?
  - — What are you declaring as your vision for the global wellness of humanity?
  - — What is your individual vision for transforming our planet, Earth?
  - — What do you see for the planet?
  - — What is your plan of action for making a difference in the world?
  - — How can your vision make the world a better place?
  - — How does your declaration improve humanity and the world?
  - — How does your vision advance our collective reality?

Examples:

— I, SupaNova Slom, see global wellness as being a place of holistic healing for the mind, body, and spirit; where our people are activated, awakened, and doing their work.

— I, Halleluyah Walcott, envision a world where collectively as humans we are focusing all our divine power to uplift both the planet and thc human race.

PART 2: SELF-ACCOUNTABILITY FOR ACHIEVING YOUR GLOBAL WELLNESS VISION

- What are you willing to do to see your vision for the global wellness of humanity manifest itself?
  - — What are your action steps for manifesting your vision?
  - — What commitments are you committing to executing and achieving for your vision to be birthed?
  - — How will you hold yourself accountable for the world to improve?

Examples:

— I, Devin, am willing to share all my skills, to share my financial knowledge, to share any knowledge that I have, and to teach what I know to those who are willing to both learn and to apply that knowledge.

— I, Wale, am willing to tame my ego, to remove competition from my nature, and to appreciate the gifts of others while sharing my own gifts. I am willing to hold myself accountable for my actions while nurturing my mind, body, and spirit as I stay in alignment.

ARIT 7: THE UNIVERSAL HUMANITARIAN MAN DAILY SPIRITUAL OBSERVANCES

ARIT POWER CENTER: PITUITARY GLAND, HAIR, SCALP, MIND, BRAIN, AND NERVOUS SYSTEM

ARIT COLOR: VIOLET

1. **THE SPIRITUAL BATH**

2. **AROMATHERAPY**

3. **YOUR ALTAR**

4. **ARIT 7 AFFIRMATION:**

   "Emancipate yourselves from mental slavery.
   None but ourselves can free our minds."

   —BOB MARLEY

5. **LIBATION**

6. **MAN HEAL THYSELF WELLNESS WARRIOR PRAYER**

7. **PITUITARY VISIONARY EMPOWERMENT AFFIRMATION—ARIT 7:**

   May my pituitary center that houses my crown, mind, hair, and scalp function in optimal wellness. May my connection with the Source of Creation assist me in uplifting and unifying humanity into harmony. May the healing of my crown reflect the abundant vitality in my pituitary as my crown reflects the abundant vitality in my higher consciousness. I envision myself and all my relations renewed in body, mind, and spirit. Throughout my lifestyle of daily purification and rejuvenation, my mind is liberated, free to create a world of humanity.

8. **CHANT (HESI)**

9. **FIRE BREATHS**

10. **HEALING STONE MEDITATION AND VISUALIZATION**

11. **HERBAL TONICS**

12. **WELLNESS WARRIOR JOURNAL WRITING**

13. **AFFIRMATION CONFIRMATION**

14. **PRAYER OF FORGIVENESS**

15. **PROBLEM-SOLVER AFFIRMATIONS**

16. **VALUE AND POWER AFFIRMATIONS**

17. **ACCOUNTABILITY POWER CHARGE AFFIRMATION CONFIRMATION**

18. **LOVE AFFIRMATIONS**

19. **COMMUNICATION AFFIRMATIONS**

20. **RESPONSIBILITY AFFIRMATIONS**

21. **EMPOWERMENT AFFIRMATIONS**

22. **INNER VOICE POWER CHARGE AFFIRMATION**

23. **CROWN AFFIRMATIONS**

24. **EXERCISE: COMPLETE YOUR WORKOUT FROM THE MAN HEAL THYSELF 12-WEEK WORKOUT PLAN**

CHAPTER 7

MAN OF SELF-MASTERY

ARIT STATE 8:
THE ILLUMINATED MAN OF ENLIGHTENMENT

ARIT STATE 9:
THE HARMONIZING MAN OF SERENITY

ARIT STATE 10:
THE NATURE MAN OF REGENERATION

ARIT STATE 11:
THE ALCHEMIST MAN OF CHANGE

ARIT STATE 12:
THE SUPREME MAN OF SELF-MASTERY

"The future offers each of us significant challenges and opportunities. We can repeat our past experiences or we can explore new levels of awareness. We can chart a flight plan for success."

—BOB LAW
Chair of Million Man March,
NY Committee

A SUPREME MAN OF OPTIMAL WELLNESS

Bob Law, who stands 6 feet 5 inches tall, is a Supreme Man. He is one of my heroes. With his calm persona and velvet voice on WWRL air waves, he lifted up our community. His profound intelligence and huge heart combined with a careful approach to healing our social dilemmas with his wisdom made him not only my hero but our hero. He loves us.

It was Bob Law who encouraged me to write my first book, the little green book, *Heal Thyself for Health and Longevity*. For years, I had really wanted an opportunity to be on his radio show. Then it happened. His vibrant and beautiful wife, Muntu Law, came to me for a holistic consultation. Muntu Law and I bonded. She said her husband could also benefit from wellness support. She made an appointment for her husband to come and see me.

Once we met and he became familiar with my holistic work, Bob Law blessed me with the opportunity to be a guest on his radio show. That was the beginning of the expansion of my work in a very public way. He fully supported "liberation through purification," the concept I promote as the heart of Healing Thyself. I became a regular on his show. In 2000, I was introduced to his "circle," which gave me the opportunity to travel with them to retreats and seminars around the country, promoting our shared vision of Wellness. We even went on Wellness cruises.

In 2008, Bob Law held a Wellness seminar for Black men and those who love them. The panel of presenters included Dr. James McIntosh; Bob Law himself; his wife, Muntu Law; and me, your sister, Queen Afua. Bob Law put out an urgent call around the issue of Black men's health. He presented statistics from the New York City Department of Health that reported that African American men consistently had the highest rates of disease in almost all categories. The data covered Black populations in all the boroughs of New York City. Bob Law further stated that as we enter the 21st century, far too many Black men are dying in their late fifties and early sixties. All too often we are losing our men to poor health care, poor nutrition, and poor stress management.

Then Bob Law said, "After a decade of nurturing women, Queen Afua is fulfilling a promise she made in 1995, at the time of the Million Man March. She is turning her attention to the wellness of Black men." He gave wellness a "shout-out" as he told everybody that he had discovered a new strategy to achieve optimal health. He invited the men at the seminar to do the same. He told them what I had been saying about learning to live with Wellness instead of with avoidable pain. He told them they could learn how to protect their prostate and to cleanse their colon. They could overcome stress and get their blood pressure and diabetic conditions under control.

Bob Law, my brother, kept me close to him while he nurtured me in the process of bringing Wellness to my brothers and sisters. He compelled me to produce my Wellness formulas and make them available to a larger audience. At the seminar, Bob Law said to me, "Stick with me, kid; I'll help you reach the people with your Heal Thyself mission."

After serving the community and our people nationwide for three decades, Bob Law has retired from talk radio. He is greatly missed. I don't see Mr. Law often now, but he will forever be a part of my work. I recognize him as a Supreme Man because of his commitment to helping me grow my vision and restore our people to wholeness. During the 1960s and 1970s, Bob Law believed that our right to wellness was a critical part of the Civil Rights Movement. He was then and continues to be an activist for Wellness.

The following segment of Man Heal Thyself Wellness Warrior takes you on the quest to awaken the super powerful, super brilliant you. Tap into a holistic, high frequency of living as you evolve into an Illuminated Man of Enlightenment. Nurture the Nature Man within as you learn to commune with nature. Become the Alchemist Man who transforms himself and others from a deadly lifestyle to a lifestyle of Wellness. Claim your joy and prosperity as you become the Supreme Man of Self-Mastery.

ARIT 8: THE ILLUMINATED MAN OF ENLIGHTENMENT

> "I am that I am.
> A shining being dwelling in light"
>
> "Nuk pu nuk khu ami khu."
>
> —THE PAPYRUS OF ANI

OPENING THE WAY:

The Illuminated Man is a supreme man of radiance who sits on his inner throne of illuminating light. He is committed to his spiritual practice, recognizing the continuous spiritual nourishment that is required to maintain his enlightened way of being. He is a healer and a messenger for and of the divine. The Illuminated Man is a magnificent manifester. He possesses a oneness with the Most High; praying, meditating, affirming, and visualizing.

The Illuminated Man of Enlightenment is authentic, activated, awakened, and aligned. He consistently nurtures his mind, body, and spirit to remain in balance and in harmony. He flows through life like water. He adapts and transforms willingly and unabashedly.

The Illuminated Man has transcended his ego, realizing insecurities and self-doubts are all constructions of negative thoughts, not the essence of his true being. He pours into himself and into others with love, compassion, empathy, mercy, and praise. He rises above jealousy, rage, inferiority, domination, and oppression, as these are all social constructs created from the ego, not from love and compassion.

The Illuminated Man is mindfully aware of the importance of living in the present and embracing the here and now. He receives all the blessings and lessons that his journey provides for him with unconditional love and acceptance. He receives knowledge, insights, realizations, and remedies from his life's blessings and lessons. He forgives himself and all others for past mistakes and misgivings. The Illuminated Man has overcome.

The Illuminated Man breaks toxic habits and patterns that have been created from karmic debt. He does not place blame. The Illuminated Man takes full responsibility and accountability for what he attracts. He seizes each opportunity to grow, expand, and learn from his life's experiences.

The Illuminated Man lives from a place of awareness, witnessing and observing. He pays attention to the synchronicities and messages that he receives from the natural world. He is connected to and in tune with Mother Nature and the energy of the cosmos.

The Illuminated Man sees the light at the beginning, middle, and end of the tunnel. He is a seeker of truth, guiding others into the light and encouraging them to shine brilliantly like he shines. The Illuminated Man is in the world but not of the world. He is a shining being dwelling in light and love.

"This little light of mine, I'm going to let it shine."

—UNKNOWN

Freedom Song

PROTECT YOURSELF:

Wellness Salute, Beloved Brother! The work we are doing right now is so very important. We—you, me, and our brotherhood—must protect ourselves. Our preservation is of the utmost priority. We must stay on our wellness game. We are healing. We are fine-tuning. We are holistically transforming mind, body, and spirit. We are tapping into both our divine masculine and divine feminine. We are releasing our light into the world. We are balanced. We are activated. We are awakened. We are aligned. We are standing strong in our power with our alpha minds, living life through a wellness vision of the highest order. We are Wellness Warriors! We protect ourselves and all our relations!

The signal we send out into the universe will define how we are received by the universe, so pay attention to the energy being emitted. Strengthen your signal to reflect your alpha state, dear brother. The universe will affirm whatever is being signaled. What we think will attract the kind of world we live in. How we carry ourselves will invite how we are perceived. We must be the light!

We command that our spirits, minds, and bodies are shielded from the adverse energies within us and outside of us. We command that our speech and utterances be divine reflections of our thoughts in action for optimal living. The moment we declare our blessed revelations, we will encounter oppositional forces propelled to challenge our pronouncements. So, daily, we must protect our sacred words. For our protection, our commitment to our daily commitments is crucial. Our daily commitments are our shields of protection. We are shielding ourselves from our own egos and from our adversaries. When we dive deeper into our pledge to ourselves and to our Fraternity of Wellness, our shields of protection are stronger and mightier.

We are affirming ourselves. We know our names. We are here. We receive fully. We are problem-solvers. We are holding our heads to the sky. We are keeping our signals on high. We are staying on our seats of power as kingsmen, as builders, as fathers, as brothers. We are receiving our responsibilities.

We must also fortify and spiritually protect all our relationships. When we make a declaration to another, part of that proclamation is committing to daily rituals to protect that relationship. If the commitment is not there from everyone involved, the relationship will be sacrificed. For the relationship to function optimally, each person must confirm and affirm their daily commitments to oneself and to the other. So, beloved brother, our commitments to ourselves must be signed, sealed, and delivered daily through our rituals for self-mastery and for spiritual fortification. As examples, we are showing and proving what that commitment through daily action looks like when the alphas affirm themselves. In our relationships, when we work together with one another, we are unified, balanced, and shielded.

As we dial in on the nuances, fine-tune the disciplines, master our wellness rituals over time, we become authentic living examples of enlightened men. We shine like the sun, who does not dim its light for anything or anyone. We shine brightly!

PART 1: PLEDGE OF ILLUMINANCE

- Create a personal Pledge of Illuminance that declares how you will no longer dim your light moving forward.
  - —What are you declaring to the world for you to shine brightly?
  - —How can you exist in a world where your light is bright?
  - —How do you radiate?
  - —How do you shine?

ARIT 8: THE ILLUMINATED MAN DAILY SPIRITUAL OBSERVANCES

AS A SUPREME MAN OF RADIANCE, I SIT ON MY INNER THRONE OF ILLUMINATING LIGHT

1. **THE SPIRITUAL BATH**

2. **AROMATHERAPY**

3. **YOUR ALTAR**

4. **ARIT 8 AFFIRMATION:**

   "Keep my head to the sky
   For the clouds to tell me why."

   —EARTH, WIND & FIRE

5. **LIBATION**

6. **MAN HEAL THYSELF WELLNESS WARRIOR PRAYER**

7. **EMPOWERMENT AFFIRMATION:**

   May my brain and higher mind, which house my mind, inner throne, and higher Aritu, function in optimal wellness. May my mind not be imbalanced, confused, or clouded. May I be on my inner throne now and forevermore. With each breath that I take, I affirm my power and my purpose. May all my visions be actualized through the clarity of my seeing. May I release all that is no longer serving me. May my mind, heart, and inner sun be in harmony and oneness. May I maintain attunement with my ancestors and the Most High. May I ascend to new heights as I radiate the highest vibration of Ma'at and divinity.

8. **CHANT (HESI)**

9. **FIRE BREATHS**

10. **HEALING STONE MEDITATION AND VISUALIZATION**

11. **HERBAL TONICS**

12. **WELLNESS WARRIOR JOURNAL WRITING**

13. **AFFIRMATION CONFIRMATION**

14. **PRAYER OF FORGIVENESS**

15. **PROBLEM-SOLVER AFFIRMATIONS**

16. **VALUE AND POWER AFFIRMATIONS**

17. **ACCOUNTABILITY POWER CHARGE AFFIRMATION CONFIRMATION**

18. **LOVE AFFIRMATIONS**

19. **COMMUNICATION AFFIRMATIONS**

20. **RESPONSIBILITY AFFIRMATIONS**

21. **EMPOWERMENT AFFIRMATIONS**

22. **INNER VOICE POWER CHARGE AFFIRMATION**

23. **CROWN AFFIRMATIONS**

24. **EXERCISE: COMPLETE YOUR WORKOUT FROM THE MAN HEAL THYSELF 12-WEEK WORKOUT PLAN**

ARIT 9: THE HARMONIZING MAN OF SERENITY

> "I live in right and truth. I am pure of heart within a pure body."
>
> —THE PAPYRUS OF ANI

OPENING THE WAY:

The Harmonizing Man is cool, calm, and collected. He is true to himself. He honors his purpose and his greatness. He knows himself. He embraces his Godhead with peace and love. The Harmonizing Man lives in gratitude. He gives thanks for all his blessings and lessons that have created the narrative of his journey. He accepts his narrative with unconditional love for himself and for all who he has encountered and interacted with, for he knows he would not be the man he is in this moment without all his blessings and lessons.

The Harmonizing Man accepts what is, without judgment. He views life without resistance. He recognizes what he can and cannot change. The Harmonizing Man leads from his heart. He is compassionate and empathetic. He is thoughtful and kind. He is forgiving and patient. He is humble and gracious.

The Harmonizing Man is in alignment with his words, thoughts, feelings, and actions. He is mindful of what he says, what he does, what he feels. He responds with acceptance and love instead of ego and judgment.

The Harmonizing Man experiences an inner and outer sense of peace.

His mind, body, and soul are in balance. He practices self-discipline. The Harmonizing Man is in supreme harmony with humanity. He can evoke unity with his fellow humans, both man and woman. He emanates cooperation and goodwill with family, friends, community, coworkers, and all his relations. He inspires, influences, and energizes those who are out of balance to transform into congruence.

The Ancient Afrakan term for harmony is Ma'at, the cosmic order that permeates all creation. Ma'at represents balance, truth, righteousness, order, law, propriety, and reciprocity. Spirituality, government, relationships, and professions are based on the principles of Ma'at, represented by the feather. The heart is seen as the seat of intelligence. The heart is weighed with the feather of Ma'at on the scale, one against the other, as shown in the judgment scenes on the walls of many Egyptian temples.

If the heart is maintained in balance with the feather on the scale, then harmony with life is achieved, for the heart would be equal to the lightness of NTR, the One Most High. The Harmonizing Man's heart is light as a feather.

ACCEPTANCE AND COURAGE:
Wellness Salute, King! We—you, me, and our brotherhood—are a family. We are actively deployed in our Wellness together. We are connected. We are connecting. We are energizing, charging, and electrifying each other and ourselves. We are bringing balance and harmony to ourselves, to each other, and to all our loved ones. We are establishing the tones and setting the examples. We are equipped. We are glowing.

We are living in the present and are committed to the right here, right now. We are cultivating our value daily. We are receiving ourselves fully, as today is what we have. Now is the beginning of all tomorrows. So, we are not judging ourselves by our past, by our successes, or by our failures. We are owning who we are in this very tangible and powerful moment.

We are letting go of our egos. We are surrendering. We are trusting the Most High. We are activating and awakening the spirits within us to flow with peace and faith. We are unifying our minds, bodies, and spirits through acceptance and courage. We are being consistent with our holistic rituals and staying committed to our commitments. We are reassessing, resetting, reprogramming, rejuvenating, restoring, and renewing. Our words, actions, and deeds are edifying and professing our power as kings.

When we affirm ourselves daily, we are demonstrating self-discipline, humility, gratitude, and dominion over our lives. We are using words of affirmation to empower ourselves. We are vibrating serenity, courage, and wisdom when we tap into our inner consciousness through our daily affirmations. We are giving ourselves the opportunity to know and to engage with our higher selves. By declaring who we are in the words that we choose to use to ourselves and to others, we recognize and command our sovereignties. All our relationships act as complements to that recognition of our value and power. Our relationships are reflections of who we are.

The goal of our Wellness Journey is to achieve self-mastery, to be the greatest and best versions of ourselves daily. To achieve this optimum wellness, we must accept and take responsibility for our value and worth each and every day. We must put the work into ourselves to heal and to release. We must exercise to build and to move. We must have the tenacity to transform. Our Wellness Journey is a marathon. To reach the finish line, we must have endurance and fortitude. Our affirmations are our reminders to maintain and to sustain our strength. Our affirmations assist us in our abilities to manage our mental and emotional spaces as we navigate the complexities of life. The repetitious act of affirming ourselves is part of our training to achieve harmony and balance. Our affirmations become our strength to move us forward at our most optimal levels. Our affirmations build us up. Our affirmations encourage us to keep going. Our affirmations remind us of who we really are.

When we arrange the way for ourselves, we are calling in our higher selves. Our Godheads are being announced. We are claiming our divine order. We are wearing our highest crowns. We are renewing ourselves to sit on our thrones, to stand on our centers, and to be our boldest, bravest, and most courageous selves.

Dear Brother! Steel sharpens steel! Love yourself! Love your people!

Declare yourself! Declare your people! Speak your truth! Speak your power!

Live in balance! Live in harmony! Live in Ma'at! Unify!

ACCEPTANCE AND COURAGE ASSIGNMENTS:

PART 1: 9 POWER COMMANDMENTS OF HARMONY AND SERENITY

- Create 9 tenets that you declare for yourself and for your brothers to achieve harmony and serenity.
  - What 9 things do you need to master each day to achieve harmony and serenity?
  - What are 9 powerful charges to live by to achieve harmony and serenity daily?
  - What are your 9 salutes of power to receive harmony and serenity in your life?

PART 2: POWERFUL MUHAMMAD ALI CHARGES

- Listen to/watch 2 or 3 Muhammad Ali speeches and/or interviews.

"It's the repetition of affirmations that leads to belief. And once that belief becomes a deep conviction, things begin to happen."

—MUHAMMAD ALI

American Professional Boxer, Activist, and Philanthropist

ARIT 9: THE HARMONIZING MAN DAILY SPIRITUAL OBSERVANCES

AS A SUPREME MAN OF BALANCE, I SIT ON MY INNER THRONE OF HARMONY

1. **THE SPIRITUAL BATH**
2. **AROMATHERAPY**
3. **YOUR ALTAR**

4. **ARIT 9 AFFIRMATION:**

   "I live in right and truth.
   I am pure of heart within
   A pure body."
   —*The Papyrus of Ani*

5. **LIBATION**

6. **MAN HEAL THYSELF WELLNESS WARRIOR PRAYER**

7. **EMPOWERMENT AFFIRMATION:**

   May my brain and higher mind, which house my mind, inner throne, and higher Aritu, function in optimal wellness. May my mind not be imbalanced, confused, or clouded. May I be on my inner throne, now and forevermore. With each breath that I take, I affirm my power and my purpose. May all my visions be actualized through the clarity of my seeing. May I release all that is no longer serving me. May my mind, heart, and inner sun be in harmony and oneness. May I maintain attunement with my ancestors and the Most High. May I ascend to new heights as I radiate the highest vibration of Ma'at and divinity.

8. **CHANT (HESI)**

9. **FIRE BREATHS**

10. **HEALING STONE MEDITATION AND VISUALIZATION**

11. **HERBAL TONICS**

12. **WELLNESS WARRIOR JOURNAL WRITING**

13. **AFFIRMATION CONFIRMATION**

14. **PRAYER OF FORGIVENESS**

15. **PROBLEM-SOLVER AFFIRMATIONS**

16. VALUE AND POWER AFFIRMATIONS
17. ACCOUNTABILITY POWER CHARGE AFFIRMATION CONFIRMATION
18. LOVE AFFIRMATIONS
19. COMMUNICATION AFFIRMATIONS
20. RESPONSIBILITY AFFIRMATIONS
21. EMPOWERMENT AFFIRMATIONS
22. INNER VOICE POWER CHARGE AFFIRMATION
23. CROWN AFFIRMATIONS
24. PROTECTION AFFIRMATIONS
25. GRATITUDE AFFIRMATIONS
26. ANCESTOR AFFIRMATIONS
27. POWER AFFIRMATIONS
28. DIVINE INTENTION AFFIRMATIONS
29. REGENERATION AFFIRMATIONS
30. EXERCISE: COMPLETE YOUR WORKOUT FROM THE MAN HEAL THYSELF 12-WEEK WORKOUT PLAN

ARIT 10: THE NATURE MAN OF REGENERATION

> "Golden are my limbs, blue my crown,
> emerald my body."
>
> —THE PAPYRUS OF ANI

OPENING THE WAY:

The Nature Man lives in cooperation with nature. He is in tune and in sync with the cosmos and the natural elements. He acts in accordance with the laws of nature and the laws of the universe. He honors the equilibrium of nature and the tranquility it provides to his mind, body, and spirit. The Nature Man lives in harmony with the clockwise movement of the universe as well as the flow of wellness, wholeness, and balance.

The Nature Man is directly connected to Source. He is energetically aligned. He observes and receives the messages, synchronicities, and downloads being communicated by the natural world. He converses with the Air (wind), Fire (sun), Water (oceans, rivers, lakes, waterfalls), and Earth (trees, plants, mountains, grasslands). He is within nature and nature is within his High Supreme Consciousness. The Nature Man trusts in nature for the opportunity to drink, bathe, wash, eat, and consume the life force of divinity.

The Nature Man is a medicine man, sharing his gifts with himself as well as others. He has knowledge of the natural elements. He applies his insight of air, fire, water, and earth to restore, to rejuvenate, to rebuild, and to detox from mental, physical, emotional, and social diseases. The Nature Man has a reverence for holistic healing and the African Natural Lifestyle.

The Nature Man is one with nature, living in harmony and balance with nature. He addresses all concerns and challenges with the elements in nature. He has an arsenal of natural tools to use in his healing work. He applies his knowledge of the properties of the elements to heal:

- Earth: Earth foods, vegetables, herbs, fruits, clay, sand, and soil
- Water: Water-rich foods, waterfalls, lakes, rivers, oceans, rain, and warm water compresses

- Fire: Fire foods, sunlight, hot springs, hot baths, and steams
- Air: Air foods, raw live foods, wind, and breathing

Just as the master botanist George Washington Carver communed with plants to bring healing to humanity, so does the Nature Man. Just like Imhotep, the father of medicine, transformed and healed with the forces of nature, so does the Nature Man. The Nature Man embraces the mantra Man Heal Thyself.

PREPARED AND EQUIPPED:

Wellness Salute, King! We—you, me, and our brotherhood—are inspiring and motivating each other. We are working together. We are fueling each other and ourselves to forge ahead on our wellness path to self-mastery. As we continue to climb our ladders of ascension, we must be prepared and equipped. Doing the work means preparing the way and clearing the space to enter the world with our tools in hand. As we climb higher and higher up the ascension ladder, we will face challenges and obstacles that want to knock us down and throw us off balance. We will not allow that to happen! We are mighty and resilient! We are tenacious and determined!

We are moving in forgiveness, love, and compassion. No longer are we asking. Instead, we are declaring. We are pouring into ourselves and releasing all that no longer serves us. We are clearing the way for our salvation and elevation. We are sitting on our thrones. We are standing in our divine power. We are wearing our crowns. We are prosperous, powerful Black kings. We are medicine men. We are pioneers. We are revolutionaries. We are the first line of honor. We are vibrant, healthy, and unified.

As we pour into ourselves, we bless ourselves. As we love ourselves as divine beings on Earth, we enthrall others. Our queens anoint us. Our brothers anoint us. As we uplift and raise ourselves out of stagnation and mediocrity, we electrify our beloved ones to do the same. We are the conduits for vitality. Our relationships are now our personal restoration-ships. We are complements of each other. We restore, rejuvenate, regenerate, and renew each other.

No longer are we operating out of obligation or a need for approval. We are implementing out of connection, purpose, and intention. We are divinely anointed by the cosmological womb of the Almighty. We are moving differently. We are seeing differently. We are thinking differently. We are returning to our truth and to our power. We have faith in the Most High. We have guidance from our ancestors. We have support from our spirit guardians. We are tapped in. We are activated, aligned, and awakened. We are growing spiritually, mentally, physically, emotionally, and energetically. We are humble and grateful.

We are establishing our longevity. We are becoming aware. We are trusting ourselves. We are using our intuitions and our instincts. We are adding to our toolboxes. We are navigating from the heart space with openness and reciprocity. We are applying the knowledge we are gathering into action. We are creating balance. We are holding ourselves accountable. We are taking responsibility. We are engaging at our highest and wisest. We are consistent. We are committed. We are showing up 100 percent. We are Wellness Warriors!

"Say it loud: I'm black and I'm proud!
Say it loud: I'm black and I'm proud!"

—JAMES BROWN

American Singer, Songwriter, Dancer,
Musician, Record Producer, and Bandleader

PREPARED AND EQUIPPED ASSIGNMENTS:

PART 1: DECLARATION OF REJUVENATION AND RESTORATION

- Create a Declaration of Rejuvenation and Restoration that identifies and affirms the nourishment you need as a king to remain empowered on your throne of natural living.
  - — What are you willing to affirm and to commit to in order to rejuvenate and restore yourself?
  - — How will you salute your personal power through regeneration?
  - — How do you operate?
  - — What is necessary daily for you to be nourished in order to honor yourself?
  - — What do you need to be at your most optimal level?
  - — What nourishment do you need as a king sitting on your power of natural living?
  - — What do you need to reaffirm?
  - — How will you regenerate yourself so that your natural light shines and every relationship is a complement to your highest self?

Examples:

— I, SupaNova Slom, am declaring my rejuvenation and restoration. The nature of me is to move in my highest mind. The nature of me is to move in my God mind. At this moment, I will stay hydrated. I will seed my rituals. I will take my baths. I will execute my altar work. I will not miss a day without affirming myself. I will do the work daily.

— I, Mentchu Ma'at, am a firestorm upon this planet. It is by way of fire I bring forth heightened states of consciousness. All the elements are at my disposal. My mission is already in motion. My mission is already complete. My actions will echo in eternity. By way of fire, we all purify and will be purified. From the ashes of our lower selves may we be rejuvenated.

PART 2: WATER CHARGE

- Spend time near a body of water.
- Let the body of water praise and celebrate you.
- Let the body of water restore and rejuvenate you.

ARIT 10: THE NATURE MAN DAILY SPIRITUAL OBSERVANCES

AS A SUPREME MAN OF NATURE, I SIT ON MY INNER THRONE OF NATURAL LIVING

1. **THE SPIRITUAL BATH**

2. **AROMATHERAPY**

3. **YOUR ALTAR**

4. **ARIT 10 AFFIRMATION:**

   "Golden are my limbs,
   Blue my crown,
   Emerald my body."
   —*The Papyrus of Ani*

5. **LIBATION**

6. **MAN HEAL THYSELF WELLNESS WARRIOR PRAYER**

7. **EMPOWERMENT AFFIRMATION:**

   May my brain and higher mind, which house my mind, inner throne, and higher Aritu, function in optimal wellness. May my mind not be imbalanced, confused, or clouded. May I be on my inner throne, now and forevermore. With each breath that I take, I affirm my power and my purpose. May all my visions be actualized through the clarity of my seeing. May I release all that is no longer serving me. May my mind, heart, and inner sun be in harmony and oneness. May I maintain attunement with my ancestors and the Most High. May I ascend to new heights as I radiate the highest vibration of Ma'at and divinity.

8. **CHANT (HESI)**

9. **FIRE BREATHS**

10. **HEALING STONE MEDITATION AND VISUALIZATION**

11. **HERBAL TONICS**

12. **WELLNESS WARRIOR JOURNAL WRITING**

13. **AFFIRMATION CONFIRMATION**

14. **PRAYER OF FORGIVENESS**

15. **PROBLEM-SOLVER AFFIRMATIONS**

16. **VALUE AND POWER AFFIRMATIONS**

17. **ACCOUNTABILITY POWER CHARGE AFFIRMATION CONFIRMATION**

18. **LOVE AFFIRMATIONS**

19. **COMMUNICATION AFFIRMATIONS**

20. **RESPONSIBILITY AFFIRMATIONS**

21. **EMPOWERMENT AFFIRMATIONS**

22. **INNER VOICE POWER CHARGE AFFIRMATION**

23. **CROWN AFFIRMATIONS**

24. **PROTECTION AFFIRMATIONS**

25. **GRATITUDE AFFIRMATIONS**

26. **ANCESTOR AFFIRMATIONS**

27. **POWER AFFIRMATIONS**

28. **DIVINE INTENTION AFFIRMATIONS**

29. **REGENERATION AFFIRMATIONS**

30. **EXERCISE: COMPLETE YOUR WORKOUT FROM THE MAN HEAL THYSELF 12-WEEK WORKOUT PLAN**

ARIT 11: THE ALCHEMIST MAN OF CHANGE

"On this day I am reborn. I am purified."
—THE PAPYRUS OF ANI

OPENING THE WAY:
The Alchemist Man is an elevated man of nature and spirituality. He is magical and mystical. He is confident and self-assured. He is grounded simultaneously in reality and spirituality. He is able to harmoniously influence the physical and vibrational worlds within him as well as outside of him.

The Alchemist Man stands comfortably in his own light. He shines brightly, emitting dynamic rays of power and energy. He holds himself and others in integrity from his heart and from his spirit. He celebrates change.

The Alchemist Man is a potent transformer. He possesses the ability to move and transmute energy in people, places, and things through his thoughts, actions, and deeds. He offers a different perspective, envisioning possibilities and solutions. He relishes the power of constructive change, empowering others to be their most magnificent.

The Alchemist Man makes a difference quickly. He cultivates his gifts of metamorphosis through his mobility. He transforms negative into positive. He transmutes toxicity into purity. He converts a challenge into an opportunity. He transforms disease into wellness. He transmutes darkness and gloom into light and beauty. He shifts a defeated person into an inspired soul. The Alchemist Man moves energy to higher ground.

The Alchemist Man trusts his greatness. He is a beacon for truth and enlightenment, guided by his intuition and his instincts. He continuously bears witness to the power of the Most High because of his unflinching devotion and faith. He channels directly from Source, allowing his creativity and artistry to flow. He believes in miracles. He trusts in the laws of the universe. He *overstands* that he is one and whole with all. Just as he can transform himself, he can do so with all things.

The Alchemist Man transcends fear and impossibilities. He believes that anything is achievable. He is a powerful manifester. When he creates an intention, he knows he will birth this intention into reality. The visions from his mind's eye produce brilliant fruit for him.

TRANSMUTE:

Wellness Salute, Victorious! We—you, me, and our brotherhood—are the catalysts for change! We are practicing the art of transmutation. We are balanced, grounded, and present. No longer are we allowing our emotions and our egos to get the better of us. No longer are we acting out of trauma, rage, anger, hurt, insecurities, or self-doubts. Instead, we are using the practices of a holistic lifestyle to maintain harmony within as well as outside of ourselves. We are mindful and aware. We are committed to our commitments every single day. We are navigating from a place of love, open to receive and give in return. We are living in gratitude and in appreciation. We are humbled and honored by all our blessings and all our lessons.

We accept and respect change, as change is constant and ever expanding. No longer are we resistant to change, as change is inevitable. Change is unavoidable. We welcome the possibilities that come with new beginnings. We release. We let go. We practice non-attachment. We are better versions of ourselves today than we were yesterday, as change offers an opportunity for rebirth. We celebrate our renewal by seizing the moment with intention.

As we love ourselves unconditionally, we are learning to embrace who we are completely with kindness and generosity. We accept our feelings fully without them possessing us. We see our emotions as an opportunity for curiosity and growth. We ask ourselves pointed questions about our feelings. We dive deep into the relationships we have with our emotions. As we heal, we gain clarity, peeling away our layers of hurt, trauma, rage, anger, insecurities, and self-doubts. We learn to accept the complexities of being human. We forgive. We release. We let go. All from places of love. All from the heights. All from wisdom. We welcome all aspects of who we are as we stand in our power.

Though we are challenged to choose ourselves first, we recognize the importance of pouring into ourselves daily. When we choose ourselves first, we are prioritizing our healing so that we can give ourselves fully to others and can be of greatest service to others. When we do our daily mind, body, and spiritual work, we are activating and aligning. We are being distinguished men of service. We are bettering ourselves as we better others.

As we claim our sovereignties as alpha men, we use the elements of life with the intention of transformation. We apply the attributes of change to align our thoughts, actions, and deeds to empower ourselves. We set the stage for our dreams to come true. We are mighty creators. We are powerful manifesters. We birth our visions. We bring into existence the unseen from the seen.

We are divine examples of empowered men who embrace their intuitions. We value ourselves! We speak our Godheads into existence! We speak our power into existence! We speak from our hearts! We use every day to be fully expressed! We live in a declared state of being!

"It's been a long
A long time coming
But I know a change gonna come."

—SAM COOKE

American Singer, Songwriter,
Composer, Producer, and Entrepreneur

TRANSMUTE ASSIGNMENTS:

PART 1: SPIRITUAL DECLARATION OF CHANGE

- Create a Spiritual Declaration of Change that advocates how you will transmute any stressors that are affecting you physically, emotionally, and spiritually.
  — What is your call for change in this moment?
  — What are you declaring spiritually?
  — What are you feeling stressed about?
  — What blocks need releasing?

Examples:

— I, SupaNova Slom, as an Alchemist Man of Change, declare that I am cultivating my transfiguration. I am taking all the beauty of this Holy Spirit inside of me. I am bringing the Holy Spirit fully forward into my physical manifestation. My transfiguration is fully expressed. My spiritual body is fully expressed.

— I, Halleluyah Walcott, as an Alchemist Man of Change, declare that my old self is no more. My transfiguration is currently underway. My spirit is excited to see what my new form will take. The king in me feels more real than what I felt before. As though I were in a dream. I am now awake and actually living. I am shaking off the slumber of a very long sleep.

PART 2: HIGHEST AND WISEST

- As an Alchemist Man of Change, how are you able to be of service to others at your highest and wisest?
  — What does being of service to others mean to you?
  — What does being at your highest and wisest mean to you?
  — What does being an Alchemist Man of Change mean to you?

Examples:

— I, Ray, as an Alchemist Man of Change, am living proof of great victory. I exist. Love will always overflow. May anything or anyone, no matter where I am, in close or far contact, be healed and live a greater life. I am the example of divine love and holistic wellness. I am healed. And everyone shall be healed.

— I, Human, as an Alchemist Man of Change, will source light to ordinary men to be extraordinary fathers, extraordinary sons, extraordinary brothers, extraordinary partners, extraordinary friends, as well as the women who love them. As an Alchemist Man of Change, transforming the space within me inspires others to transform from energy to architecture. As an Alchemist Man of Change, I vibrate higher today than I did yesterday to transmute fear into love. As an Alchemist Man of Change, we are surrendered. All boats rise because we choose courage over comfort. We embrace our roles as healers and healed.

ARIT 11: THE ALCHEMIST MAN DAILY SPIRITUAL OBSERVANCES

AS A SUPREME MAN OF POWER, I SIT ON MY INNER THRONE OF TRANSFORMATION

1. **THE SPIRITUAL BATH**

2. **AROMATHERAPY**

3. **YOUR ALTAR**

4. **ARIT 11 AFFIRMATION:**

   "On this day, I am reborn.
   I am purified."
   —*The Papyrus of Ani*

5. **LIBATION**

6. **MAN HEAL THYSELF WELLNESS WARRIOR PRAYER**

7. **EMPOWERMENT AFFIRMATION:**
   May my brain and higher mind, which house my mind, inner throne, and higher Aritu, function in optimal wellness. May my mind not be imbalanced, confused, or clouded. May I be on my inner throne, now and forevermore. With each breath that I take, I affirm my power and my purpose. May all my visions be actualized through the clarity of my seeing. May I release all that is no longer serving me. May my mind, heart, and inner sun be in harmony and oneness. May I maintain attunement with my ancestors and the Most High. May I ascend to new heights as I radiate the highest vibration of Ma'at and divinity.

8. **CHANT (HESI)**

9. **FIRE BREATHS**

10. **HEALING STONE MEDITATION AND VISUALIZATION**

11. **HERBAL TONICS**

12. **WELLNESS WARRIOR JOURNAL WRITING**

13. **AFFIRMATION CONFIRMATION**

14. **PRAYER OF FORGIVENESS**

15. **PROBLEM SOLVER AFFIRMATIONS**

16. **VALUE AND POWER AFFIRMATIONS**

17. **ACCOUNTABILITY POWER CHARGE AFFIRMATION CONFIRMATION**

18. **LOVE AFFIRMATIONS**

19. **COMMUNICATION AFFIRMATIONS**

20. **RESPONSIBILITY AFFIRMATIONS**

21. **EMPOWERMENT AFFIRMATIONS**

22. **INNER VOICE POWER CHARGE AFFIRMATION**

23. **CROWN AFFIRMATIONS**

24. **PROTECTION AFFIRMATIONS**

25. **GRATITUDE AFFIRMATIONS**

26. **ANCESTOR AFFIRMATIONS**

27. **POWER AFFIRMATIONS**

28. **DIVINE INTENTION AFFIRMATIONS**

29. **REGENERATION AFFIRMATIONS**

30. **EXERCISE: COMPLETE YOUR WORKOUT FROM THE MAN HEAL THYSELF 12-WEEK WORKOUT PLAN**

ARIT 12: THE SUPREME MAN OF SELF-MASTERY

> "I have made an end of my failings.
> I have made the way."
>
> —THE PAPYRUS OF ANI

OPENING THE WAY:

The Supreme Man is the supreme elevated man. He stands tall and confident wearing his crown of supreme consciousness. He is the creator of his own reality, for he knows who he is at his most pure and authentic essence. He is self-aware. He is in total oneness with his whole state of being. He trains and practices daily to maintain and to protect the harmony and balance he has achieved through his wellness journey. The Supreme Man vibrates at the highest levels of optimal wellness.

The Supreme Man understands that to maintain his highest level of optimal wellness, his life is a continual exploration of advancing his mind, body, and spirit. As he moves forward, he is in a continual process of knowing himself, creating himself, growing himself, improving himself, transcending himself, and maintaining himself.

The Supreme Man leads with his heart. He is guided by love and light. He creates his present and future selves through his visions, thoughts, actions, deeds, and affirmations. He realizes his potential and allows his ego to get out of the way. The Supreme Man lives in the moment, right here, right now, without attachment. By being present, he connects with his highest and wisest self through divine oneness with Source and supreme consciousness. He surrenders willingly and without resistance.

The Supreme Man is courageous and brave. He chooses to actively overcome his trials and tribulations of pain, suffering, and dis-ease. He chooses to sit in his discomfort to heal and to release the weight of the heavy baggage that he has been carrying that no longer serves him. The Supreme Man rises out of the mud, rebirthing himself, to become Nefer Atum, the lotus blossom of highest consciousness. He transforms as he navigates the 12 states of man's inner journey, using the waters of life's lessons to purify and elevate himself.

The Supreme Man radiates inner and outer beauty. He emanates light and oneness for all to enjoy. He shines brightly and stands comfortably in his own light with humility. He is an example of liberation, empowerment, and transcendence.

The Supreme Man is a leader of humanity. He vibrates at the highest frequencies known to man. Through his awakening, the world is restored.

ACTIVATED:

Wellness Salute, my Mighty and Powerful Brother! We—you, me, and our brotherhood—celebrate you as we celebrate ourselves standing tall in our supreme consciousness of wellness. You have activated your seat of self-mastery! You have risen out of the mud and blossomed! You have committed to your commitments! You have poured into yourself daily! You have overcome any challenges and obstacles that you have encountered along your journey to wellness. You have healed. You have released. You have forgiven. You have affirmed. You have embraced and accepted the essence of who you are.

Yet, dear brother, your wellness narrative does not stop here. In fact, you are only just beginning. We are only just beginning. As we declare ourselves Supreme Men of Self-Mastery, we must protect our crowns. At this moment, this turning point, you will be confronted by your ability to maintain your activated seat of self-mastery. The universe will support you, but the universe will also test you. So, it is time to dive deeper into your healing, realizing that self-mastery is a never-ending responsibility of growth, change, and development. Self-mastery is a process of becoming. Self-mastery is practice and dedication. Great brother, how will you stay authentic to yourself? What are you willing to do to maintain your activated seat of self-mastery? What are you willing to do to protect your activated seat of self-mastery? What are you willing to do to strengthen your activated seat of self-mastery? How will you continue to enhance your inner God? How will you continue to fortify your inner God? How will you continue to energize your inner God?

We are alpha men of action! We are master problem-solvers! We are medicine men! We are Wellness Warriors! We are prepared and equipped. We navigate with confidence. We are committed to our commitments. We pour into ourselves daily. We love ourselves unconditionally. We use words of power to uplift and energize. We forgive. We release. We let go. We move forward.

Our minds are clear. Our energy is focused. Our souls are awakened. We are elevating. We are ascending. We are activated. We are unstoppable. We are unified. So be it. So it is. Wellness Salute, Victorious! **Asé!**

> "The game is gonna test you, never fold.
> Stay ten toes down. It's not on you, it's in you and what's in you, they cannot take away."
>
> —NIPSEY HUSSLE
>
> *American Rapper, Activist, and Entrepreneur*

ACTIVATED ASSIGNMENT:

PART 1: SUPREME MAN OF SELF-MASTERY DECLARATION

- Create a Supreme Man of Self-Mastery Declaration that describes who you are as a Supreme Man of Self-Mastery.
  - What does being a Supreme Man of Self-Mastery mean to you?
  - Who are you at the essence and core of your being?
  - Who are you at your highest and wisest?
  - How are you empowering yourself?
  - How do you see yourself from this moment on, forever?
  - How do you embody and embrace your activated seat of power of supreme consciousness of wellness?

PART 2: OPERATION PROTECT THE SUPREME MAN OF SELF-MASTERY DECLARATION

- Create a Protection Declaration that illustrates how you will protect and strengthen your seat of power daily.
  - What are you willing to do to protect and strengthen your seat of power daily?
  - How will you stay authentic to yourself and protect your authenticity daily?
  - How will you continue to enhance, fortify, and energize your inner God?
  - How will you use your wellness tools to defend your crown?
  - How will you prepare for war or deployment in and through life's uncertainties?
  - How will you remember to protect yourself through your spiritual rituals and affirmation confirmations?
  - How committed are you to continuing to activate your plant medicines and plant-based nutrition for

continued growth and development without excuses, distractions, or procrastination?

PART 3: AFFIRMATION CONFIRMATION REVISIT

- Review the affirmation you wrote at the beginning of Arit 1: The Family Man of Unity and Wealth.
- Revise your Affirmation Confirmation. Go deeper into your healing by strengthening your inner God power with words that energize, electrify, motivate, and fortify your highest consciousness.

PART 4: PRAYER OF FORGIVENESS REVISIT

- Review the Prayer of Forgiveness you revised in chapter 5, Arit 4: The Lover Man of Harmony.
- Revise your Prayer of Forgiveness again. Go deeper into your healing. Allow yourself to feel and acknowledge what you need to forgive within yourself so your heart opens and shines brightly.
- Hold yourself accountable while releasing self-judgment and self-criticism.

PART 5: RETURN TO THE FOUNDATION

- Go within, sit in conversation with yourself, and reflect about your journey to self-mastery so far.
- Spend time identifying the growth you have achieved as you navigated through each of the Arits during this particular self-healing journey.
- How did you transform?
- What did you release?
- What did you shed?
- Who are you now?
- What blockages remain?
- What traumas and pains remain?
- How will you dive deeper into your healing?

- Return to Arit 1: The Family Man of Unity and Wealth, and begin the next level of your healing to strengthen and motivate your movement forward.

ARIT 12: THE SUPREME MAN DAILY SPIRITUAL OBSERVANCES

AS A SUPREME MAN OF WELLNESS, I SIT ON MY INNER THRONE OF PHYSICAL, MENTAL, AND SPIRITUAL SELF-MASTERY

1. **THE SPIRITUAL BATH**
2. **AROMATHERAPY**
3. **YOUR ALTAR**
4. **ARIT 12 AFFIRMATION:**
   "On this day, I am reborn.
   I am purified."
   —*The Papyrus of Ani*
5. **LIBATION**
6. **MAN HEAL THYSELF WELLNESS WARRIOR PRAYER**
7. **EMPOWERMENT AFFIRMATION:**
   May my brain and higher mind, which house my mind, inner throne, and higher Aritu, function in optimal wellness. May my mind not be imbalanced, confused, or clouded. May I be on my inner throne, now and forevermore. With each breath that I take, I affirm my power and my purpose. May all my visions be actualized through the clarity of my seeing. May I release all that is no longer serving me. May my mind, heart, and inner sun be in harmony and oneness. May I maintain attunement with my ancestors and the Most High. May

I ascend to new heights as I radiate the highest vibration of Ma'at and divinity.

8. **CHANT (HESI)**
9. **FIRE BREATHS**
10. **HEALING STONE MEDITATION AND VISUALIZATION**
11. **HERBAL TONICS**
12. **WELLNESS WARRIOR JOURNAL WRITING**
13. **AFFIRMATION CONFIRMATION**
14. **PRAYER OF FORGIVENESS**
15. **PROBLEM-SOLVER AFFIRMATIONS**
16. **VALUE AND POWER AFFIRMATIONS**
17. **ACCOUNTABILITY POWER CHARGE AFFIRMATION CONFIRMATION**
18. **LOVE AFFIRMATIONS**
19. **COMMUNICATION AFFIRMATIONS**
20. **RESPONSIBILITY AFFIRMATIONS**
21. **EMPOWERMENT AFFIRMATIONS**
22. **INNER VOICE POWER CHARGE AFFIRMATION**
23. **CROWN AFFIRMATIONS**
24. **PROTECTION AFFIRMATIONS**
25. **GRATITUDE AFFIRMATIONS**
26. **ANCESTOR AFFIRMATIONS**
27. **POWER AFFIRMATIONS**
28. **DIVINE INTENTION AFFIRMATIONS**

29. REGENERATION AFFIRMATIONS

30. EXERCISE: COMPLETE YOUR WORKOUT FROM THE MAN HEAL THYSELF 12-WEEK WORKOUT PLAN

ON MY INNER THRONE

As a Supreme Man of Self-Mastery, I sit on my inner throne of optimal body, mind, and spiritual wholeness. He is the man who actively overcomes his trials and tribulations of pain and suffering. A man who vibrates and lives to his optimal frequency. Out of the mud of trials and tribulations, pain and suffering, to the optimal Nefer Atum, is a man who has transformed through the waters of life lessons and has purified himself, thereby elevating himself out of the mud of man through the 12 states of man's inner journey.

The Supreme Man of Self-Mastery is the ultimate, elevated man. He is totally in oneness and aware of his complete and whole state of being. The Supreme Man is one who rebirthed himself out of the mud of *dis*ease, pain, and suffering and has therefore liberated himself through purification acts of wellness. The Supreme Man is one who has blossomed into a Nefer Atum—A Lotus Man of inner and outer beauty. The Supreme Man has the communication of all 11 Aritu from 1 through 11.

The Supreme Man of Self-Mastery is in divine oneness with higher consciousness, and he is living the highest frequency known to man. Through the Supreme Man's awakening, the world is restored.

WHAT WILL PARADISE BE FOR THE SUPREME MAN OF OPTIMAL WELLNESS?

In the Islamic faith, it is said that if a man lives a righteous Muslim life, when he goes to the afterworld, he will enter into *paradise* and have beautiful virgins as his reward. Before his transition, world-renowned Supreme Historian John Henrik Clarke used to say, "Paradise is between a black woman's thighs." As the Velvet Sword, I say this to you, Supreme Man of Optimal Wellness, "You have come into your higher self and reflect the God in you. You reflect Neter, Jah, Allah, Jehovah, Krishna, Yahweh, Jesus, Olodumare. And so, the more you purify your body, mind, and spirit, the more you will attract unto yourself a woman who embodies paradise within herself."

It is true that some men attempt to experience *paradise* with a woman while they themselves are not living a holistic life. On the other hand, if a man is a seeker of true paradise, he will strive to elevate himself beyond the wounded man and use his inner strength to become a Wellness Warrior. Courageously, he will continue his quest to become the Supreme Man of Optimal Wellness. His wellness will be his first reward of many.

You, Supreme Man of Wellness, should look forward to meeting, face-to-face, a sacred woman, a purified woman, a mystic woman, a radiant whole woman. She will be someone who shares with you: peace, not war; joy, not pain; balance, not revenge; and beauty instead of the ugliness in life. She will be sweet to taste, lovely to touch, and will emanate a most divine aroma from her body and essence from her spirit.

This woman of paradise—your inner vision of delight—will spring from the garden of your mind and spirit and heart. You will share with each other luscious and tasty vegan foods, greens, herbs, live juices, and pure water. She is free from physical disease and emotional toxicity. Your bliss will shine in and from your relationship like a million shining stars, because together you create and share a fulfilling lifestyle. This woman of paradise is energetic and wise and radiant. You share the path of wellness and are a divine reflection of consciousness and each other. You meet in the paradise that you have each created from within. Together you will conceive and birth a new world of divine order, of paradise on Earth. Heaven.

CHAPTER 8

THE EXPANDED MAN

Congratulations, Wellness Warrior!

This is a remarkable time in your life, filled with profound transformation. Throughout the reading of this book and/or having participated in our rites of passage training, you have been embarking on a journey of self-discovery that brings immense change and growth. You have been witnessing incredible revelations, tapping into the strength of your spirit, and navigating through transitions and transformations. The events that have transpired in this time have all been instrumental in leading you to this moment of awakening—an opportunity to truly understand and embrace what you deserve, gain invaluable knowledge, and prepare for the future that lies ahead.

Not only have you been rebuilding yourself from within, but you have also persevered in the face of unforeseen challenges. You have learned the art of transmuting energy and extracting meaningful life lessons from every experience. Your triumphs, though some may have unfolded in the depths of your inner world, have shaped you into the person you are today.

Even now, as you move forward, this moment remains pivotal. Take the time to reflect and listen to the calling that guides you. Find solace within yourself, allowing your inner voice to grow louder and clearer, revealing your true purpose. Remember that nobody else can live, feel, and experience your unique gift. It is you who must center yourself and forge that deep inner connection. Embrace the beautiful times that await you, both in the present and the future.

WELLNESS WARRIOR SALUTE

WELLNESS WARRIOR (((RU)))!!!

I AM SACRED, NOT SAVAGE

YOU WILL SURVIVE. YOU CAN RECLAIM YOUR DIVINITY OVER TRAUMA.

In a world plagued by hardships and adversity, it is essential to remember that our experiences do not define us but rather shape us into resilient beings. Trauma and the struggle for survival can leave lasting scars in every part of your well-being. However, it is in these moments that we have the opportunity to embrace our sacredness and reclaim our divinity. By recognizing our inherent worth and power, we can transcend the labels society may impose on us and cultivate a sense of self that is rooted in strength, healing, and empowerment.

To reclaim our divinity, we must first acknowledge the sacredness that resides within us. Regardless of our past experiences, we are born with an inherent worth and innate goodness. By recognizing this truth, we can break free from the chains of self-doubt and reclaim our intrinsic value as human beings. It is through self-acceptance and self-love that we begin to heal and rise above the challenges that life presents.

Society often labels as victims those who have endured trauma and survived. However, it is essential to move beyond this narrative of victimhood and reclaim our power. While our experiences may have shaped us, they do not define us. By embracing our strength and resilience, we can rewrite our personal narratives and shift the focus from what happened to us to how we have triumphed over adversity.

Reclaiming our divinity requires embracing a journey of healing. Healing is a deeply personal process that involves acknowledging our pain, seeking support, and engaging in practices that nurture our well-being. Whether it be therapy, meditation, creative expression, or connecting with nature, each step we take toward healing is an act of reclaiming our divine essence. And instead of allowing our past to dictate our present and future, we can make conscious choices that align with our values and aspirations. By setting boundaries, pursuing our passions, and surrounding ourselves with positive influences, we reclaim our power and establish ourselves as the architects of our own destiny.

In a world that often perpetuates a narrative of victimhood, it is crucial to remember that we are not defined by our trauma or the challenges we have faced. Instead, we are sacred beings with the power to transcend our circumstances and reclaim our divinity. By acknowledging our inherent worth, embracing our journey of healing, and cultivating empowerment, we can rise above the limitations imposed on us and create lives filled with meaning, purpose, and joy. Remember, you are sacred, not savage, and your ability to reclaim your divinity is a testament to your strength and resilience.

32 AFFIRMATIONS FOR EMBRACING YOUR DIVINE SACRED BEING

Repeat these affirmations daily to reinforce your connection to your divine sacred being and to reclaim your divinity over trauma and survival.

1. I am a unique expression of the divine, worthy of love and respect.
2. I trust in the wisdom and guidance of the sacred within me.
3. I am connected to the infinite source of love and light.
4. I embrace my inner power and use it to create positive change in the world.
5. I am a vessel of divine love, radiating love to myself and others.
6. I honor the sacredness of my body and treat it with love and care.
7. I release all limitations and open myself to unlimited possibilities.
8. I am deserving of abundance in all areas of my life.
9. I am grateful for the blessings that flow into my life.
10. I forgive myself and others, releasing any heaviness from my heart.
11. I trust in the divine timing of my life's journey.
12. I am guided by intuition and make choices aligned with my highest good.
13. I am a co-creator with the universe, manifesting my dreams into reality.
14. I embrace my unique gifts and share them with the world.
15. I let go of fear and step into a space of courage and empowerment.
16. I am surrounded by loving and supportive beings in both the physical and spiritual realms.

17. I honor the interconnectedness of all beings and treat them with kindness.
18. I am a beacon of light, inspiring others with my words and actions.
19. I trust in the divine plan for my life, even in times of uncertainty.
20. I release the need for control and surrender to the flow of life.
21. I am worthy of love, joy, and all the blessings that come my way.
22. I embrace my divine purpose and live it with passion and authenticity.
23. I am a channel for divine healing energy, bringing comfort and restoration.
24. I listen to the whispers of my soul and follow my inner guidance.
25. I release all self-doubt and embrace my inherent worthiness.
26. I am a magnet for miracles and synchronicities.
27. I radiate peace and harmony from the depths of my being.
28. I honor the sacredness of every moment and live fully in the present.
29. I am a co-creator of a world filled with love, compassion, and unity.
30. I trust that everything I need is already within me.
31. I am a divine sacred being, worthy of all the blessings that the universe has to offer.
32. I am deeply loved and supported by the divine in every aspect of my life.

PRAYER OF PROTECTION AND STRENGTH

Divine Spirit, I humbly come before you
to seek your protection and strength
for my body, this sacred temple that houses my soul.
I ask for your loving presence to surround me and shield me from harm.
Grant me the strength to nurture and care for my body,
to make choices that honor its well-being.
Help me to embrace a lifestyle that promotes
health, balance, and vitality.
Guide me toward nourishing foods, exercise, and restful sleep
so that I may thrive in body, mind, and spirit.
I ask for protection from any physical ailments or diseases
that may threaten my well-being.
May you fortify my immune system, empower my cells
to function optimally, and restore any imbalances within me.
Shield me from harm, both seen and unseen, and keep me safe
from accidents, injuries, and harm's way.
Fill this sacred vessel with your healing light,
purifying it from negativity, stress, and tension.
Help me release any burdens or worries I may carry,
allowing me to experience a state of inner peace and tranquility.

Grant me courage and resilience in the face of
adversity,
allowing me to overcome any challenges that
come my way.
Strengthen my body, mind, and spirit
so that I may navigate life's journey with grace
and determination.
May my body be a vessel for divine love, wisdom,
and compassion.
Help me to use it as an instrument to serve others,
to uplift and inspire those around me.
May my actions, words, and thoughts reflect the
sacredness within me,
radiating love and light to all beings.
I surrender my body to your divine guidance,
trusting that you will protect and strengthen it.
Thank you, Dear Spirit, for your unwavering love
and support.
With gratitude in my heart,
I embrace the prayer of protection and strength
for my body, this sacred temple.
AMEN, ASE, SHALOM, TUWA, AND SALAAM

21 AFFIRMATIONS FOR SELF-MASTERY AND EXPANSION

Repeat these affirmations regularly and believe in their power to transform your mindset and empower you on your journey of self-mastery.

1. I am capable of achieving greatness.
2. I am in control of my thoughts and emotions.
3. I believe in my abilities to overcome any challenge.
4. I am worthy of success and happiness.
5. I embrace change and use it to grow stronger.
6. I am resilient and bounce back from setbacks.
7. I trust my intuition and make wise decisions.
8. I take responsibility for my actions and their outcomes.
9. I am disciplined and committed to my goals.
10. I am open to learning and expanding my knowledge.
11. I am confident in expressing my authentic self.
12. I attract positive experiences and people into my life.
13. I radiate love and compassion toward myself and others.
14. I prioritize self-care and nurture my mind, body, and soul.
15. I forgive myself for past mistakes and embrace self-growth.
16. I let go of comparison and focus on my own journey.
17. I am fearless in pursuing my dreams and aspirations.
18. I celebrate my achievements, no matter how small.
19. I have a clear vision of my future and take steps to manifest it.
20. I surround myself with supportive and uplifting individuals.
21. I am a master of my own destiny and create the life I desire.

21 PROTOCOLS OF TRAINING TO WAGE AND WIN THE WAR WITHIN

1. Embrace self-reflection: Regularly examine your thoughts, beliefs, and actions to foster personal growth.
2. Practice empathy: Seek to understand and relate to the experiences and perspectives of others.
3. Cultivate gratitude: Appreciate the blessings and opportunities in your life, no matter how small.
4. Embody authenticity: Be true to yourself and express your thoughts and feelings honestly.
5. Foster self-compassion: Treat yourself with kindness and understanding during challenging times.
6. Embrace vulnerability: Allow yourself to be open and authentic, even if it feels uncomfortable.
7. Nurture emotional intelligence: Develop awareness and understanding of your emotions and those of others.
8. Challenge limiting beliefs: Question and reframe negative thought patterns that hold you back.
9. Engage in active listening: Give your full attention when others are speaking, seeking to understand rather than simply respond.
10. Practice mindfulness: Cultivate present-moment awareness and nonjudgmental acceptance of your thoughts and experiences.
11. Cultivate forgiveness: Release resentment and grudges, freeing yourself from emotional baggage.
12. Foster healthy relationships: Surround yourself with supportive and positive individuals.
13. Engage in self-care: Prioritize activities that promote your physical, mental, and emotional well-being.
14. Seek growth and learning: Continuously expand your knowledge and skills through education and personal development.

15. Embrace change: Embrace uncertainty and view it as an opportunity for growth and adaptation.
16. Take responsibility for your actions: Acknowledge your mistakes and learn from them, striving to make amends when needed.
17. Practice nonjudgment: Avoid making hasty assumptions about others and instead approach them with openness and understanding.
18. Cultivate resilience: Develop the ability to bounce back from setbacks and overcome challenges.
19. Foster a growth mindset: Embrace the belief that your abilities and intelligence can be developed through dedication and effort.
20. Embody integrity: Align your actions with your values and uphold ethical standards in all aspects of your life.
21. Share your wisdom: Pay it forward by sharing your experiences and insights to inspire and support others on their healing journeys.

30 AFFIRMATIONS FOR EXPANDED TRANSFORMATION

Repeat these affirmations daily, allowing them to empower and guide you on your journey of personal growth and transformation.

1. I am worthy of love, success, and abundance in all areas of my life.
2. I embrace my authentic self and honor my true desires and aspirations.
3. I am strong, resilient, and capable of overcoming any challenges that come my way.
4. I release any limiting beliefs that no longer serve my highest good.
5. I trust my intuition and make decisions that align with my soul's purpose.
6. I am open to receiving guidance and support from the universe and divine energies.
7. I am deserving of healthy and fulfilling relationships in my life.
8. I forgive myself and others, freeing myself from the burdens of the past.
9. I embrace change as an opportunity for growth and self-improvement.
10. I am confident in my abilities and trust in my own unique talents and skills.
11. I attract positivity and abundance into my life effortlessly.
12. I am committed to my personal growth and continuously evolving into my best self.
13. I am deserving of self-care and prioritize my physical, mental, and emotional well-being.
14. I release any need for control and surrender to the flow of life.

15. I am a magnet for success and attract prosperous opportunities into my life.
16. I am grateful for all the lessons I have learned and the wisdom I have gained.
17. I radiate love, kindness, and compassion toward myself and others.
18. I let go of fear and step into my power with confidence and courage.
19. I am worthy of abundance in all areas of my life, including finances.
20. I trust in the divine timing of my life's journey and embrace patience and perseverance.
21. I am committed to healing and transforming any past wounds or traumas.
22. I am open to receiving love and support from others, allowing myself to be vulnerable.
23. I attract into my life positive and uplifting people who support my growth.
24. I am connected to my inner wisdom and make decisions that align with my higher self.
25. I release any self-doubt and embrace my greatness and unlimited potential.
26. I am deserving of success and celebrate my achievements with gratitude.
27. I embrace my masculine energy with balance, honoring both strength and vulnerability.
28. I am a source of inspiration and empowerment for myself and others.
29. I release any need for perfection and embrace myself as a work in progress.
30. I am a divine being, and my personal growth and transformation have a positive impact on the world.

DEPLOYED AFTER TRAINING

COMMITMENT AND DISCIPLINE DURING EXPANSION

Embarking on a journey of self-care and personal growth requires dedication, commitment, and discipline. The Wellness Warrior represents someone who has undergone self-care training and has reintegrated into their daily life newly prepared to sustain their healing process. Key strategies and mindset shifts can support the Wellness Warrior in staying committed and disciplined while balancing the responsibilities of everyday life.

1. **EMBRACE SELF-COMPASSION:** Recognize that setbacks and challenges are a natural part of life, and it's essential to treat oneself with kindness and understanding. Instead of berating yourself for not being perfect, embrace self-compassion as a powerful tool to bounce back from setbacks and stay motivated.

2. **SET REALISTIC GOALS:** Break down your healing journey into smaller, manageable steps that align with your current life responsibilities. Doing so can help you avoid feeling overwhelmed and increase your chances of success. Remember that progress is often a gradual process, and even the smallest steps forward are still moving you in the right direction.

SMALLER STEPS:

a. If you do not have an hour for your meditation/visualization, then commit to 10 minutes at the start of your day.
b. If you do not have an hour or more to go to the gym to do physical training, allot yourself 15 minutes at home or on your job during your break to do 3 sets of push-

ups and jumping jacks to failure, and conclude with a light stretch. This protocol will engage the whole body.

c. Take 5 to 10 minutes daily to journal your thoughts and your emotions, which also allows you to read on your own. This exercise serves as a litmus test for you to check in with yourself and problem-solve the issues you need to work on.

3. **ESTABLISH CONSISTENT SELF-CARE PRACTICES:** Consistency is key when it comes to self-care. Develop a routine that incorporates various self-care practices such as exercise, meditation, journaling, and engaging in hobbies that bring you joy. Prioritize self-care by scheduling it into your daily or weekly routine, treating it as nonnegotiable time for your well-being. By making self-care a habit, you reinforce your commitment to healing.

4. **PRACTICE MINDFULNESS:** Mindfulness is a powerful tool for staying present and grounded amid life's responsibilities. By practicing mindfulness techniques like deep breathing, body scans, or mindful eating, you can cultivate awareness of your thoughts, emotions, and physical sensations. This awareness allows you to respond to stressors and challenges with clarity and intention rather than reacting impulsively.

5. **SEEK SUPPORT AND ACCOUNTABILITY:** Navigating the complexities of life while prioritizing self-care can be challenging. Surround yourself with a supportive network of friends, family, or a therapist who can provide guidance and encouragement. Share your goals and progress with them, allowing them to hold you accountable. Joining support groups or online communities with individuals

who share similar journeys can also provide valuable insights and motivation.

6. **PRACTICE TIME MANAGEMENT:** Balancing healing and life's responsibilities requires effective time management. Identify your priorities and allocate time accordingly. Learn to say no to commitments that don't align with your healing goals, creating space for self-care and personal growth. Break tasks down into manageable chunks, delegate when possible, and establish boundaries to protect your time and energy.

7. **CELEBRATE MILESTONES AND PROGRESS:** Acknowledge and celebrate milestones and progress along your healing journey. Recognize the effort and growth you have accomplished, no matter how small. Celebrating these victories reinforces your commitment and boosts motivation to continue on the path of self-care and healing.

GOD TIME VS. DEMON TIME

ACTIVATE YOUR GODHEAD TO OVERCOME PERSONAL DEMONS

In the journey of self-discovery, we all face internal struggles—our personal demons. Negative traits, such as self-doubt, fear, and destructive behaviors, can obstruct our potential. We hold the power to transcend the challenges and activate our Godhead, representing our divine potential. The contrast between God Time and Demon Time is pivotal.

While journeying toward self-discovery and personal growth, individuals often encounter internal struggles—our personal demons, the inner conflicts and negative aspects of ourselves that hold us back from reaching our full potential. Demon Time can manifest as negative thoughts and self-doubt and emotional burdens and fear, caused by destructive addictions and behavioral patterns that hinder our progress. Often these demons stem from past traumas and limiting conditioning and negative beliefs that we have internalized over time. Ignoring the existence of our internal demons hinders our progress to access and celebrate our quality of life. The time we spend denying (blindly or consciously) our personal demons are hours better spent facing them and challenging ourselves to open the pathway to our divine state of being. In the journey from Demon Time to God Time, we reach toward our Godhead to overcome personal demons and unlock our true potential. By embarking on the journey of self-discovery, cultivating self-awareness, and harnessing our inner divinity, we can triumph over negative thought patterns, destructive behaviors, and emotional burdens. Identifying our demons is the first step toward confronting them and manifesting our sacred in-dwelling God Time.

God Time embodies a higher consciousness where we connect with our true selves, which are our divine essence. In God Time, we gain the clarity of our inherent divinity. It is a state of heightened awareness and connection to universal wisdom and love. By embracing God Time, we access the strength, resilience, and transformative potential needed to overcome our personal demons.

To activate the Godhead and conquer personal demons, follow these key steps:

1. **SELF-AWARENESS:** Recognize your personal demons through honest introspection. Assess this awareness by regularly reflecting on your thoughts, feelings, and behaviors. Journaling or seeking feedback from trusted friends can help you identify patterns and gain clarity.

2. **ACCEPTANCE AND COMPASSION:** Embrace self-acceptance and show compassion toward yourself. Recognize that your demons are learned behaviors, not flaws.

3. **MINDFULNESS AND MEDITATION:** Practice mindfulness and meditation to quiet your mind and observe your thoughts without judgment. This enhances self-awareness and empowers conscious choices.

4. **POSITIVE AFFIRMATIONS AND VISUALIZATION:** Use affirmations and visualization to reprogram your subconscious, counteracting negative influences and reinforcing your Godhead potential.

5. **SEEK SUPPORT:** Build a support system through therapy, coaching, or mentoring for guidance and encouragement.

As you tap into your Godhead and embark on the journey of conquering personal demons, you will begin to experience profound transformation, leading to a life filled with purpose, growth, and fulfillment.

a. Growth and fulfillment: Transcending your personal demons opens you to personal growth and fulfillment. You become better able to cultivate healthy relationships and live a life aligned with your values and aspirations honored.
b. Empowerment: By recognizing your inherent divinity, you reclaim your power and become an active participant in your personal journey to self-mastery. You no longer feel helpless or at the mercy of your personal demons, but rather you develop a sense of agency and control over your life.
c. Liberation: Overcoming personal demons leads to lib-

eration from self-imposed limitations. You experience increased freedom, resilience, and a sense of inner peace. You embrace new possibilities and expand your horizons.

Remember, your God Time is always in reach, from *within*, empowering you to conquer your demons and celebrate your continuous extension and embrace your divine essence.

DISCOVERING YOUR PERSONAL SUPER MAN

Who is a Super Man? As an extended Wellness Warrior, you already embody your Super Man. What is a Super Man? Super Man is a principle—symbolizing immense power and godlike abilities that dwell in every young boy even before manhood. As little boys, you are pushed to go beyond your limits and become high achievers in life's ever-changing landscape. You are encouraged and sometimes even forced to become a titan in your field or even a variety of fields chosen by you or not chosen by you. You're encouraged to "Buff up!," "Buck up!," "Run!," "Jump!," "Lift!," Exceed!," "Get the highest grade!" If you fail or fall or get hurt, you're chastised, "Don't cry." Your role models have been family members, educators, entrepreneurs, athletes, artists, and scientists . . . all who have been acknowledged as being the best in their field.

Furthermore, throughout history, humanity has been captivated by tales of extraordinary individuals who possess exceptional abilities and use them for the greater good. These individuals often are referred to as superheroes. Among them, the legendary figure of Superman stands out as being the strongest, fastest, most powerful, the BEST. He is that, and that is his authenticity. Now, Wellness Warrior, this is your authenticity, you are divine. Super Man is a principle within the divinity of man in his natural state. Wellness Warrior, as you continue your journey toward self-mastery, you are encouraged to embrace and develop your indwelling BEST, your Super Man. Your purpose as a Super Man is not merely to develop your abilities for personal strength and gain but to become a protector, serving humanity as a force for justice in an often chaotic world. You bear the weight of being an example of safeguarding and expanding yourself to be at your best.

Living up to the expectations of a Super Man is not without sacrifices. Driven to prioritize the greater good over his own desires, he is prone to experiencing isolation and loneliness. Frequently, the Wellness Warrior may find himself torn between his need to establish boundaries in personal relationships as he honors his duty to expand his self-care. This suffering may separate him from the very lives and relationships he is striving to protect and inspire. Let your struggles remind you of the importance of resilience, selflessness, and the pursuit of a purpose greater than yourself.

The Super Man serves as a reminder that even the most powerful among us bear our own burdens. This principle teaches us that with great power comes not only responsibility, but also the opportunity to make a profound difference in the world.

WELLNESS WARRIOR ANIMAL SPIRITS: THE GORILLA AND FALCON

Within nature are abundant sources to remind us that all in existence is divine. The animal kingdom is filled with remarkable beings that consistently demonstrate the incredible yet attainable attributes of divinity. Two notable creatures, the gorilla on land and the falcon in the air, stand out as examples of strength, agility, and resilience—which could inspire humans to embrace their inner warrior spirit and lead balanced lives.

The gorilla is one of the strongest animals on land. With its robust physique and energetic prowess, a gorilla has the ability to lift heavy objects with ease. In their natural habitat, with their predominantly vegetarian diet added to consistent exercise, gorillas demonstrate Warrior Wellness. Furthermore, despite their massive size, gorillas display a calm demeanor and maintain a harmonious existence within their social groups.

Observing gorillas teaches us valuable lessons about daily wellness care for humans. Balancing physical strength and emotional calmness is critical, whether it be at work, while maintaining healthy relationships, or when managing our emotions. The gorilla's balanced nature reminds us of the significance of equilibrium. Just as with gorillas, incorporating strength and balance can lead us to physical and emotional well-being.

The falcon, often referred to as the "king of the skies," embodies the spirit of agility and adaptability. These magnificent birds possess exceptional aerial skills and unmatched speed, allowing them to maneuver effortlessly through the air. Their agility teaches us the importance of staying nimble in the face of life's challenges. Moreover, the falcon's keen eyesight serves as a metaphor for the importance of clarity and foresight. Falcons possess exceptional visual acuity, enabling them to spot prey from great distances. By developing flexibility, both physically and mentally, we can adapt to changing circumstances and overcome obstacles with grace. This attribute inspires us to cultivate a clear vision for our lives and set meaningful goals. With a focused mindset and a clear vision, we can navigate our paths with purpose and achieve personal growth and fulfillment.

Let the gorilla and falcon be our guides, reminding us that we, too, embody the spirit of extended Wellness Warriors.

ABOUT (((RU)))

Chanting or sounding (((RU))) is channeling the powerful warrior tones made by African silverback gorillas, found in the great forests of eastern, central, and western Africa. African silverback gorillas are the largest primates on Earth and represent strength. Imagine the sound when they (((RU))).

The Nile Valley Guardian/God of Ascension is represented by the Falcon, one that rises above. The letters RU are part of the Guardian's name, HRU/HERU. Imagine the sound of (((RU))) when chanting the name HRU/HERU.

When you are going through daily rites-of-passage challenges and/or growth and development, invoke the spirit animal tones of the warrior silverback and holy falcon. Chant (((RU)))!!! Take three deep breaths then chant (((RU))) ten to twenty times. Repeat three times a day for full wellness warrior activation.

CHANNELING SEXUAL ENERGY INTO CREATIVE LIFE FORCE

FROM SEX TO SUPER CONSCIOUSNESS

Sexuality is a powerful and innate aspect of human nature, deeply intertwined with our physical, emotional, and spiritual well-being. Beyond its reproductive function, sexual energy possesses immense creative potential that can be harnessed and channeled into various areas of our lives.

Sexual energy is a potent life force that resides within each individual. It encompasses more than mere physical desire or pleasure. It is a dynamic energy that, when consciously directed, can be transformed into a powerful creative force. Recognizing and understanding this energy is the first step toward harnessing its potential.

Rather than dissipating this energy through uncontrolled

sexual gratification, individuals can learn to channel it into more meaningful endeavors such as creativity, personal growth, and spiritual exploration. This process of redirecting sexual energy from its purely physical expression toward other aspects of life is referred to as "transmutation." Through transmutation, we can expand our consciousness and awaken our dormant potentials.

Beyond the physical and emotional realms, channeling sexual energy can lead to spiritual awakening. Various spiritual traditions emphasize the importance of sexual energy in the path to enlightenment. Techniques such as tantra, meditation, and breathwork enable individuals to harness their sexual energy, elevate their consciousness, and experience states of super consciousness. This integration of sexuality and spirituality can result in profound personal transformation and a heightened sense of connection with the divine. When approached with mindfulness and respect, sexual encounters within a loving partnership can deepen emotional bonds, enhance communication, and foster personal growth. Indeed, intimate relationships offer a unique opportunity to explore the transformative power of sexual energy. By channeling sexual energy toward mutual connection and spiritual union, couples can embark on a journey of shared exploration and harmonious growth.

Sexual energy shares a fundamental connection with creativity. Many great artists, writers, and musicians throughout history have recognized the correlation between sexual energy and their creative output. Personally, during periods of celibacy, if I found myself sexually aroused, I would redistribute the sexual energy to creating music or to writing or physical exercise in order to recycle the energy and further my self-development. By consciously channeling sexual energy, individuals can tap into their creative wellspring, unlocking new levels of inspiration, imagination, and innovation. Recognizing the transformative potential of sexual energy can help us transcend the limitations of physical pleasure and unlock the vast reservoir of creative power within ourselves. Embracing the journey from sex to super consciousness opens up new dimensions of human experience and unlocks our true creative potential.

THE WARRIOR OF LOVE, COMPASSION, AND ABUNDANCE

In a world often plagued by conflict, scarcity, and indifference, there exists a rare breed of individuals who embody the qualities of a warrior, not in the traditional sense but as warriors of love, compassion, and abundance. These remarkable souls navigate life with an unwavering commitment to spreading love, extending compassion, and fostering abundance in every aspect of their existence. They are warriors who fight against the darkness of hatred and scarcity, armed with a profound understanding of the transformative power of love and an unyielding belief in the interconnectedness of all beings.

1. LOVE:

Love, the most potent force known to humankind, serves as the foundation for the warrior of love, compassion, and abundance. This warrior recognizes that love possesses the ability to heal wounds, bridge divides, and bring about profound transformation. They wholeheartedly embrace the concept of unconditional love, extending it not only to those close to them but also to strangers, adversaries, and even the world itself. Through their actions, they sow the seeds of love, creating a ripple effect that touches lives far and wide.

2. COMPASSION:

Compassion is the warrior's beating heart—generating love and abundance. They possess an extraordinary ability to empathize with the suffering of others, recognizing the shared humanity that binds us all. This warrior stands as a beacon of kindness and understanding, offering solace to those in pain and seeking to alleviate the burdens of others. With their compassionate presence, they inspire hope, ignite healing, and remind us all of the inherent goodness within humanity.

3. ABUNDANCE:

By operating from a mindset of abundance rather than scarcity, they understand that the universe is a vast reservoir of resources, capable of providing for the needs of all. In a world often driven by competition and hoarding, this warrior sees the potential for collaboration and generosity. They embrace the belief that there is more than enough to go around and actively work toward creating a world where abundance is accessible to all. By fostering a culture of sharing, they challenge the prevailing narrative of scarcity and inspire others to do the same.

4. RESILIENCE:

The path of the warrior of love, compassion, and abundance is not an easy one. They face numerous challenges, setbacks, and moments of doubt. However, their resilience is unwavering. Armed with an unshakable conviction in the power of love, they persist in their mission to create a better world. They draw strength from their connection to a higher purpose, remaining steadfast in the face of adversity and inspiring others to do the same.

By embodying these qualities, we can all become warriors in our own right, working together to create a world where love and abundance prevail. Let us embrace the warrior within us and join the noble quest to spread love, compassion, and abundance to every corner of the globe.

SPEAKING THINGS INTO EXISTENCE

THE POWER OF VOWELS

Language is a remarkable tool that allows us to communicate our thoughts, desires, and intentions. However, beyond its practical applications, language possesses a profound influence on our lives. I firmly believe that speaking things into existence—particularly through the power of vowels—can manifest our desires and shape our reality.

Vowels are the building blocks of language, forming the core sounds that give meaning to words. They are produced with an open vocal tract and without any significant obstruction, allowing air to flow freely. Vowels are inherently connected to our emotions and hold a unique resonance within our bodies. Each vowel has a distinct frequency that resonates with different energy centers, or chakras, within us. Vowels are indeed the fundamental elements of language, and their unique sounds can evoke profound emotional responses. I first learned about this fascinating connection through my vocal coach, affectionately known as Uncle Reggie, when I was just 10 years old. He emphasized the importance of vowel sounds in vocalization, particularly in spiritual practices. For example, the elongated "ah" in "amen" is not just a mere closing word; it signifies affirmation and connection to the divine. Similarly, the prolonged "o" in chanting "om" is believed to resonate with universal consciousness, creating a sense of unity and peace. Across various cultures, the names for God often contain extended vowel sounds, emphasizing the deep spiritual significance tied to these phonetic elements.

To delve deeper into this topic, one can explore studies in sound therapy, phonetics, and even linguistics that examine the resonance of vowels and their emotional impact. Notable research has shown how specific vowel sounds can induce relaxation and alter brainwave patterns, promoting healing and well-being. Recognizable examples include the use of chanting in meditation practices, where the repetition of vowel sounds creates a calming effect. Engaging with resources such as books on sound healing or studies on the relationship between sound and emotion can further illuminate how vowels shape our communication and inner experiences. By understanding the vibrational power of these sounds, we can tap into a deeper connection with ourselves and the world around us.

The principle of speaking things into existence is rooted in the power of intention and manifestation. By deliberately vocalizing our desires and affirmations, we send out vibrations into the universe that align with our intentions. This process involves using positive, present-tense statements to reinforce a belief in the desired outcome. When we speak with conviction and clarity, our words become a powerful force that can shape our reality.

EXAMPLES:

"I AM A WELLNESS WARRIOR."
"I AM A GOOD MAN."

To effectively speak things into existence, one must cultivate a deep belief in the power of intention and the possibility of manifesting desires. Our subconscious mind plays a crucial role in this process since it holds our core beliefs and conditioning. By harnessing the vibrational power of vowels and consciously reprogramming our subconscious through repetitive affirmations, we can align our beliefs with our spoken intentions, creating a harmonious resonance that attracts what we desire and shapes our reality in alignment with our intentions. While our intentional practice may not guarantee immediate results, self-talk and mastering your inner voice can serve as a powerful tool for personal growth and transformation, allowing us to be active participants in creating our optimal reality.

OVERCOMING PERSONAL BLOCKS AND TRAUMA TO ACHIEVE SUCCESS

The journey toward personal success is often hindered by the presence of inner obstacles, unresolved traumas, and the shadow self—the hidden aspects of our personality that we may consciously or unconsciously suppress. Navigating these shadows and overcoming personal blocks and trauma are transformative processes that pave the way for self-growth, resilience, and ultimately, success. By shedding light on our shadows, embracing vulnerability, and engaging in healing practices, we can unlock our true potential and create a path toward personal and professional fulfillment.

The shadow self, a concept introduced by Swiss psychologist Carl Jung, refers to the parts of our psyche that we tend to ignore or repress, often due to societal norms or personal discomfort. This includes traits like jealousy, anger, and insecurity, as well as emotions stemming from past experiences that we consider undesirable, such as shame or guilt. For example, you might repress your anger, leading to passive-aggressive behavior or feelings of resentment. If these shadows remain unacknowledged, they can manifest as self-limiting beliefs—such as thinking "I am not worthy"—or destructive patterns that hinder personal growth. Yet, by approaching our shadows with self-compassion and curiosity, we can uncover valuable insights about our true selves and foster a more integrated identity.

To confront and heal personal blocks, it is first essential to identify and address underlying wounds. Suggested methods of identifying underlying wounds might involve seeking professional help, such as therapy, or engaging in introspective practices including journaling and mindfulness (a type of meditation in which you focus intensely on what you are sensing and feeling in the moment, without interpretation or judgment). A friend of mine found immense clarity through art therapy, where expressing his feelings through painting allowed him to confront past traumas and understand the blocks that were holding him back from overcoming his shadows. By excavating and comprehending our personal blocks, we can begin to dismantle their influence on our lives, creating a pathway for healing and growth.

Navigating the shadow self involves embracing our vulnerabilities and engaging in deep self-reflection. This process involves having difficult conversations with ourselves about our fears, insecurities, and past mistakes—essentially confronting the parts of ourselves that we often avoid. Vulnerability, in this context, means being open and honest about our struggles, which creates a safe space for personal growth. The role of another person, such as a therapist or trusted friend, is crucial in this exploration; their support and perspective can help us feel less alone in our journey, encouraging us to dig deeper and face uncomfortable truths without judgment.

Self-reflection, on the other hand, is a solitary endeavor where we assess our thoughts and feelings independently. This can be exemplified through practices like journaling, meditation, or quiet contemplation, which allow us to process our emotions and experiences. Reflective practices yield clarity about our core values, aspirations, and the recurring patterns that hinder our progress. By actively engaging in these practices, we support the healing warrior within us, fostering a deeper understanding of ourselves. This newfound awareness helps us clearly identify the areas where we need growth, as it outlines the proactive steps necessary for meaningful personal development. Through this committed self-exploration, we pave the way for a more authentic and fulfilling life.

20 REMEDIES FOR NAVIGATING THE SHADOW SELF

This list can provide a starting point to help you navigate your shadow self and overcome personal blocks and trauma for success.

1. Embrace self-reflection: Take time to explore your thoughts, emotions, and past experiences to uncover your shadow self.
2. Practice self-compassion: Be kind and patient with yourself as you navigate through challenging emotions and memories.
3. Seek professional help: Consider working with a therapist or counselor who specializes in trauma and shadow work.
4. Develop a support system: Surround yourself with understanding and supportive individuals who can provide guidance and encouragement.
5. Cultivate mindfulness: Engage in practices like meditation and deep breathing to increase self-awareness and manage stress.
6. Utilize journaling: Write down your thoughts, fears, and aspirations to gain clarity and insight into your shadow self.
7. Practice forgiveness: Let go of grudges, resentments, and self-blame to heal and move forward.
8. Set healthy boundaries: Learn to say no and prioritize your well-being, protecting yourself from toxic relationships and situations.
9. Engage in creative expression: Explore art, music, or writing to express and process your emotions.
10. Build resilience: Focus on developing coping mechanisms and strengthening your emotional resilience to face challenges.
11. Prioritize physical well-being: Make self-care activities like exercise, healthy eating, and adequate sleep important in your daily life to support your overall well-being.

12. Identify triggers: Become aware of situations or people that trigger negative emotions or memories, and develop strategies to manage them effectively.
13. Practice self-acceptance: Embrace all parts of yourself, including the shadow self, without judgment or shame.
14. Release limiting beliefs: Challenge negative beliefs that hold you back and replace them with empowering ones.
15. Engage in shadow work exercises: Explore techniques like inner child healing, guided visualization, or dream analysis to address unresolved traumas.
16. Cultivate gratitude: Focus on the positive aspects of your life and express gratitude daily to shift your mindset.
17. Seek inspiration: Surround yourself with uplifting books, podcasts, or role models who have overcome similar challenges.
18. Take small steps outside your comfort zone: Gradually expose yourself to situations that provoke fear or discomfort to expand your personal growth.
19. Celebrate progress: Acknowledge and celebrate your achievements, no matter how small, as you navigate through your healing journey.
20. Embrace ongoing self-growth: Recognize that personal growth is a lifelong process and commit to continuous self-improvement and self-discovery.

PERSONAL DEVELOPMENT AND DISCIPLINE

In an era marked by constant distractions and the pursuit of instant gratification, the importance of personal development and discipline cannot be overstated. To truly thrive in life, one must adopt the mindset of a Wellness Warrior—a person who actively seeks growth, cultivates positive habits, and exhibits unwavering discipline.

Habits play a significant role in shaping our lives. A Wellness Warrior recognizes the importance of fostering positive habits that support their physical, mental, and emotional well-being. Whether it involves regular exercise, a balanced diet, meditation, or journaling, these habits become the building blocks of a healthy and fulfilling life.

Life is rife with challenges and setbacks, and it is the ability to weather these storms that sets a Wellness Warrior apart from others. Through personal development and discipline, individuals acquire the mental resilience required to navigate difficult circumstances with grace and determination. They understand that setbacks are opportunities for growth and use them as stepping stones toward a stronger and more resilient version of themselves.

1. **FACING JOB LOSS:** Imagine someone who unexpectedly loses their job. Instead of succumbing to despair, they take this setback as an opportunity to reassess their career goals, acquire new skills, and ultimately find a job that is more fulfilling.

2. **OVERCOMING ILLNESS:** A person diagnosed with a chronic illness may initially feel overwhelmed. However, through personal development, they learn to manage their condition, seek support, and adopt a healthier lifestyle,

turning their experience into a source of strength and advocacy for others.

3. **ENDURING RELATIONSHIP BREAKUP:** After a painful breakup, an individual might focus on self-improvement, exploring their interests, and developing new friendships. This process helps them emerge stronger and more aware of what they want in future relationships.

4. **FACING ACADEMIC CHALLENGES:** A student struggling with a particular subject might experience frustration. By seeking help, studying harder, and developing better study habits, they not only improve their grades but also build confidence and resilience that will benefit them in future challenges.

5. **ASSUMING A PHYSICAL FITNESS JOURNEY:** Someone embarking on a fitness journey might face setbacks and injuries. Instead of giving up, they adapt their training regimen, learn about nutrition, and celebrate small victories, ultimately achieving their fitness goals and gaining a deeper understanding of their body's capabilities. These examples illustrate how individuals can turn challenges into opportunities for growth, embodying the Wellness Warrior mentality.

Discipline serves as the backbone of personal development. It is the unwavering commitment to one's goals and the ability to stay focused despite distractions and temptations. A Wellness Warrior understands that discipline is not merely a means to an end; it is a way of life. Through discipline, individuals cultivate consistency, perseverance, and self-mastery, enabling them to overcome obstacles and achieve their desired outcomes.

For those who have struggled to cultivate personal discipline, I can offer support and practical strategies to help them redefine their relationship with discipline. By introducing them to the teachings in *Man, Heal Thyself*, readers can gain a fresh understanding of discipline as not merely a rigid set of rules enforced in a cruel way, but as a dynamic practice that fosters self-awareness and personal growth. This book encourages men to explore the underlying motivations and beliefs that influence their behaviors, inviting them to approach discipline with compassion and patience rather than harshness. Through this lens, discipline becomes a tool for empowerment, enabling individuals to align their actions with their values and aspirations. By sharing insights and fostering a supportive community, we can inspire a transformative journey toward a more disciplined and fulfilling life.

Transformation extends beyond each individual—just as a lack of discipline may have created a lifetime of strained relationships or evaluations (at work, in fitness, or in social settings), consistent and measurable efforts toward personal development can inspire others, creating a ripple effect of positive change. By leading through example, Warriors can encourage those around them to embark on their own personal growth journeys, fostering a culture of wellness and empowerment.

WELLNESS WARRIOR ROBERT A. BAILEY SHARES HIS STORY

I became a mental health therapist for two reasons. First, to prevent others from suffering as I had, having dealt with anxiety and depression since childhood. Second, I longed for the tools to build and sustain a happy, healthy family. I believed that by learning the skills to assist others in creating strong relationships, I could also transform my own life. My journey has been one of relentless searching—seeking tools, models, and paths that could address the challenges within our community. So, when I discovered the Man Heal Thyself program developed by SupaNova Slom and co-facilitated by Halleluyah Walcott, I knew it was time to dive in. Having already encountered the profound work of SupaNova and his mother, Queen Afua, I trusted in the immense value of their wisdom.

The 12-week program was nothing short of transformative. At one point, when the group's commitment waned, SupaNova delivered a powerful correction, reminding us that complacency is the choice to decay and that our work together was a matter of life and death. He challenged us to live with a mighty (((RU)))! That moment reignited my passion for healing and rebirth. Trauma often robs us of our divine right to wellness, allowing fear and hurt to dominate. Man Heal Thyself helped me reclaim my center, rewriting myself and my care back into my narrative.

Before this program, wellness had become something I pursued to gain significance. I believed that if I healed and regained my former vitality, I would become acceptable. If I restored my energy, I could prove my worth through intellect and ability. But the program challenged this mindset: If we heal to be worthy, then how will we be worthy enough to heal? I learned that I heal because I am already sufficient. I consume the purest foods because I am already sacred. Even at my lowest, I remain beautiful and worthy.

Man Heal Thyself was rejuvenating—a special serum crafted specifically for my soul. In a world that demands we exhaust ourselves, this program was a call to slow down and remember our sacredness. To anyone considering this journey, I say: Slow down, brother. The work will always be there, but your spirit won't wait forever. Take the time to reflect, restore, and join a community of men committed to becoming Wellness Warriors in a world intent on our destruction. Healing is the great controversy of our time. Step into it with courage.

Wellness Warrior Salute,
WW Robert A. Bailey, LCSW

Ultimately, by becoming Wellness Warriors, we shape a brighter and more empowered future for ourselves and those around us.

ACTIVATION OF THE DIVINE MASCULINE

The concept of divine masculine activation refers to the awakening and realization of the inherent divine qualities found within masculine energy, such as strength, courage, assertiveness, and protection. This activation represents a dynamic exploration and embodiment of these positive aspects of masculinity, aimed at fostering balance, harmony, and authentic expression both within individuals and the collective. Historically, in various cultures, masculine energy has often been linked to dominance, aggression, and power-seeking behaviors. However, the divine masculine offers a different perspective. It encourages men to reconnect with their higher selves and true essence, embracing qualities such as compassion, integrity, vulnerability, and emotional intelligence.

Notably, this activation is beneficial not only for men but also for women and therefore for society at large. One of the key objectives of divine masculine activation is to create balance and restore harmony within relationships and communities. He strives to recognize within himself that the qualities traditionally associated with the divine feminine (such as empathy, nurturing, and receptivity) are not gender specific and are indwelling in himself as well. The divine masculine seeks to identify and develop empathy, nurturing, and receptivity within himself. This dynamic interplay of energies fosters more authentic and equitable partnerships, where masculine and feminine aspects are equally recognized and valued. By integrating the positive elements (regardless of whether branded "masculine" or "feminine"), individuals can engage in healthier and more fulfilling connections with each other and within the community.

When men embody their higher qualities, they can become agents of positive change—promoting social justice, equality, and inclusivity, and challenging outdated norms and systems that perpetuate inequality. The divine masculine also inspires leadership grounded in compassion, wisdom, and integrity, fostering a more balanced, enlightened, and sustainable world for all.

20 KEYS TO HELP UNLOCK THE DIVINE MASCULINE

UNLOCKING THE DIVINE MASCULINE IS AN ONGOING JOURNEY OF PERSONAL GROWTH AND SELF-DISCOVERY.

1. Cultivate self-awareness: Understand your strengths, weaknesses, and patterns of behavior.
2. Embrace vulnerability: Allow yourself to express emotions authentically and connect with others on a deeper level.
3. Cultivate inner strength: Develop resilience, determination, and the ability to face challenges head-on.
4. Foster healthy relationships: Practice open communication, empathy, and respect in your interactions with others.
5. Seek balance: Strive for a harmonious integration of your masculine and feminine energies.
6. Embody integrity: Act in alignment with your values, maintaining honesty and ethical behavior.
7. Practice self-care: Prioritize your physical, mental, and emotional well-being.
8. Cultivate compassion: Show empathy and kindness toward yourself and others.
9. Embrace your purpose: Discover and pursue your passions, aligning your actions with your life's mission.
10. Develop leadership skills: Inspire and empower others through clear communication, vision, and collaboration.
11. Embrace growth and learning: Continuously seek knowledge, challenge your beliefs, and expand your horizons.
12. Cultivate mindfulness: Stay present and cultivate awareness of your thoughts, emotions, and actions.

13. Practice active listening: Truly hear others without judgment, allowing them to express themselves fully.
14. Embody healthy masculinity: Reject harmful stereotypes and embrace traits such as strength, compassion, and accountability.
15. Foster healthy boundaries: Respect your own boundaries and honor those of others.
16. Embrace personal responsibility: Take ownership of your choices and actions, and learn from your mistakes.
17. Cultivate a sense of purpose: Connect with a higher meaning in life and align your actions with that purpose.
18. Cultivate self-discipline: Develop healthy habits, set goals, and follow through with commitments.
19. Embody courage: Face your fears and take bold action, even in the face of uncertainty.
20. Embrace partnership: Recognize the value of collaboration, cooperation, and shared responsibility in relationships.

CREATIVITY AND SPIRITUALITY

Creativity and spirituality share a profound and intricate connection, both serving as gateways to deeper self-expression, understanding, and transcendence. While creativity is often associated with the arts, it extends beyond that to encompass innovative thinking, problem-solving, and the ability to imagine new possibilities. Spirituality, on the other hand, refers to the exploration of one's inner self, seeking meaning, purpose, and connection to something greater than oneself.

At their core, both creativity and spirituality involve tapping into a source of inspiration that goes beyond the limitations of the rational mind. They invite us to venture into the realm of intuition, imagination, and the unseen. When we engage in creative pursuits, whether it be painting, writing, or composing music, we enter a state of flow where time seems to dissolve, and we become fully present in the moment. Similarly, spirituality invites us to be fully present and attuned to the depths of our being, connecting us to the essence of life and the universe.

Creativity and spirituality share a common ground in their ability to transcend boundaries. They enable us to break free from conventional thinking and explore new perspectives. By delving into our creative potential, we tap into the depths of our imagination, allowing us to envision new possibilities and challenge the status quo. Similarly, spirituality encourages us to question societal norms and delve into the mysteries of existence, fostering a sense of curiosity and wonder.

Both creativity and spirituality are deeply personal and subjective experiences. They allow us to express our authentic selves and connect with something greater than the individual ego. When we create, whether it be a painting or a poem, we infuse a part of our essence into the work, revealing aspects of our inner world. This act of self-expression can be deeply cathartic and healing, offering a means to connect with our emotions, thoughts, and experiences. Spirituality, too, involves a journey of self-discovery and self-expression, unraveling the layers of our being and allowing us to connect with the divine or the sacred.

Moreover, creativity and spirituality have the power to connect individuals and communities. Art, music, and literature have the ability to transcend cultural and linguistic boundaries, evoking emotions and fostering a sense of unity among diverse individuals. Spirituality, likewise, can bridge gaps and foster a sense of interconnectedness, emphasizing the shared human experience and our connection to the world around us.

The connection between creativity and spirituality is profound—both offer pathways to self-discovery, personal growth, and connection with something greater than ourselves. Engaging in creative pursuits can nurture our spiritual well-being, while exploring our spirituality can fuel our creative endeavors. Together, creativity and spirituality enrich our lives, enabling us to explore the depths of our being, express ourselves authentically, and forge connections with the world and the divine.

CONSTRUCTIVE STEPS IN CONFIDENCE AND INTERNAL STRENGTH

Confidence and self-mastery are critical components of psychological dominance for men. Achieving psychological dominance involves a deep understanding of oneself, the ability to exude confidence, and mastering the art of influence. Here are some steps for men to practice in self-mastery and confidence:

1. **SELF-AWARENESS:** Begin by understanding your strengths, weaknesses, and triggers. Reflect on your past experiences and how they have shaped your beliefs and behaviors. This

introspection helps in identifying areas for improvement and growth.

2. **MINDFULNESS AND EMOTIONAL REGULATION:** Practice mindfulness to stay present and in control of your emotions. By understanding and regulating your emotions, you can project a sense of calm and composure that is essential for psychological dominance.

3. **PHYSICAL HEALTH:** Taking care of your physical health is crucial. Regular exercise, a balanced diet, and sufficient sleep not only contribute to a healthy body but also have a significant impact on mental well-being and confidence.

4. **PERSONAL DEVELOPMENT:** Continuous learning and personal growth are fundamental to self-mastery. Engage in activities that challenge you intellectually, emotionally, or physically. This could involve learning new skills, reading, or pursuing hobbies that expand your knowledge and capabilities.

5. **EFFECTIVE COMMUNICATION:** Mastering the art of communication is key. Practice active listening, articulate your thoughts clearly, and develop the ability to convey your ideas with confidence. Effective communication is a powerful tool in asserting psychological dominance.

6. **BODY LANGUAGE:** Pay attention to your body language. Practice open, confident postures and maintain eye contact during conversations. These nonverbal cues communicate strength and assurance.

7. **GOALS:** Set realistic yet challenging goals and work consistently toward achieving them. The sense of

accomplishment from reaching milestones enhances self-confidence and reinforces self-mastery.

8. **FEARS AND RISKS:** Confronting fears and taking calculated risks are essential for personal growth. Stepping out of your comfort zone builds resilience and confidence in your abilities.

9. **POSITIVE SELF-TALK:** Cultivate a positive mindset through affirmations and constructive self-talk. Believing in your capabilities and reinforcing positive beliefs about yourself is foundational to psychological dominance.

10. **MENTORSHIP:** Surround yourself with individuals who exude the qualities you aspire to embody. Seeking guidance from mentors can provide invaluable insights and support in your journey toward self-mastery and confidence.

Achieving psychological dominance involves a holistic approach encompassing self-awareness, emotional regulation, continuous growth, effective communication, and the cultivation of a confident mindset. By consistently practicing these steps, men can develop the psychological dominance that emanates from self-mastery and confidence.

UNRAVELING THE POWERS OF THE MIND-BODY CONNECTION

In a groundbreaking discovery that challenges traditional notions of the mind-body relationship, a recent study has illuminated the intricate and inseparable link between the quality of an individual's thoughts and the biochemical processes within the body. This revelation not only sheds light on the far-reaching implications for mental and physical well-being but also underscores the potent influence of the mind over bodily functions.

Dr. Maya Patel, a leading neuroscientist at Stanford University, spearheaded the research that has sent ripples through the scientific community. "Our study unveils the remarkable interplay between mental states and biochemical activities," Dr. Patel explained. "The implications are profound, as they underscore the vital importance of nurturing positive and constructive thoughts for overall health and well-being."

The study, published in the *Journal of Neurology and Biochemistry*, delved into the intricate mechanisms through which thoughts and emotions exert tangible effects on the body's biochemistry. For instance, it was revealed that persistent negative thoughts and stress can trigger the release of cortisol, a hormone known for its adverse impact on immune function and cardiovascular health. Conversely, positive and optimistic thoughts were found to stimulate the production of endorphins and dopamine, fostering a harmonious biochemical environment conducive to overall health.

To illustrate the tangible effects of this mind-body connection, the study examined the case of John Smith, a 45-year-old executive who had been grappling with chronic stress and anxiety. Through a series of mindfulness and cognitive behavioral therapy sessions, Mr. Smith underwent a transformative shift in his thought patterns, cultivating a more optimistic and resilient mindset. Subsequent biochemical analyses revealed a notable reduction in stress-related hormones and a surge in "feel-good" neurotransmitters, mirroring his newfound mental landscape. "The changes in my thinking seemed to have a tangible impact on how I felt physically," Mr. Smith remarked. "It's truly eye-opening."

Furthermore, the study uncovered profound implications

for various health conditions, including chronic pain, autoimmune disorders, and even cancer. By homing in on the study of the mind-body connection, researchers are exploring innovative therapeutic approaches that integrate cognitive strategies with conventional medical treatments, aiming to optimize patient outcomes of quality of life.

Dr. Sanjay Gupta, a renowned psychiatrist and author, emphasized the imperative of recognizing and harnessing the powers of the mind-body connection. "We are witnessing a pivotal shift in our understanding of health and healing," Dr. Gupta stated. "By acknowledging the profound influence of thoughts on biochemistry, we open new frontiers for personalized medicine and holistic well-being."

The implications of this study are far-reaching, with potential ramifications for diverse fields ranging from health care and psychology to education and public policy. As the boundaries between mind and body continue to blur, society stands at the threshold of a new era—one that celebrates the intrinsic harmony between mental and physical well-being, ushering in a paradigm shift with transformative potential for individuals and communities alike.

In the wake of this groundbreaking research, the imperative to nurture a positive and balanced mental landscape takes on renewed significance, offering a compelling invitation to explore the depths of the mind-body connection and unlock its profound powers for the betterment of humanity.

A LETTER TO THE INCARCERATED WELLNESS WARRIOR

Recently, one of my Instagram followers, Sister Kim Dehaarte, bought 20 copies of *Man, Heal Thyself* for men currently incarcerated in Texas who are part of a men's voluntary accountability group. She reached out, asking me to write a letter of encouragement as the men voyage on their wellness journeys.

Greetings, Brothers—Wellness Warrior Salute!

I am SupaNova Slom, author of *Man, Heal Thyself: The Wellness Warrior's Journey to Self-Mastery*. In the journey of self-discovery and healing you have embarked on, I want to commend each one of you for your courage, commitment, and dedication to your growth. It takes incredible strength to confront our vulnerabilities and past traumas, and by being part of this voluntary accountability group, you have already taken a monumental step toward your own healing and transformation.

As you delve into the pages of *Man, Heal Thyself*, may you find solace, inspiration, and tools to navigate your personal journey with resilience and grace. Remember, healing is not a linear path, but a continuous evolution of self-awareness and growth. Embrace each moment, each lesson, and each challenge as an opportunity to rise stronger and wiser. Know that you are not alone in this journey. Together, as a community of Wellness Warriors, you have the power to uplift, support, and inspire one another toward greater self-mastery. Your commitment to healing not only transforms your own lives but also ripples out to positively impact those around you.

Stay strong, stay dedicated, and never underestimate the power of your own resilience. You are capable, you are worthy, and you are deserving of all the love and healing that comes your way.

With deep respect and admiration for your strength,

SupaNova Slom

CHAPTER 9

WE SPEAK

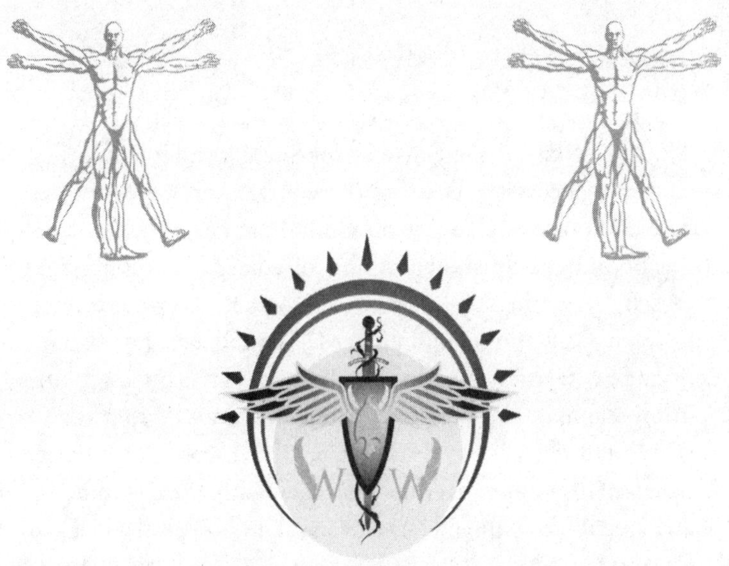

THE
WELLNESS WARRIOR
SHIELD

"If you wanna make the world a better place
Take a look at yourself, and then make a change."

—MICHAEL JACKSON
August 29, 1958—June 25, 2009

(Man Heal Thyself thanks you, MJ,
a global healing visionary.
All praises.)

TESTIMONIALS & STATEMENTS

FROM WELLNESS WARRIOR GRADUATES OF MAN HEAL THYSELF RITES OF PASSAGE

KNOW MYSELF, LOVE MYSELF

I am forever grateful to the MOST HIGH, the SUPREME INTELLIGENCE of the Universe for SupaNova Slom and Halleluyah Walcott for creating the content for the Man Heal Thyself book as well as the program. I can't express how much this book has helped me not only dive deeper into improving myself by getting to know myself better, accepting myself, loving myself, and rebuilding my self-confidence, but also fortifying my relationship with my Wife as well as my loved ones in my Cipher. The best part about this book is that it's for every man regardless of race, age, creed, status, or religious beliefs. This book is very much needed within our community and I highly recommend it to anyone. This book is the ideal gift for your Husband, Father, Brother, Son, Uncle, Cousin, Nephew, Boyfriend, or Male Friend. So, if you're reading this testimonial, it means you've made the right decision to take the steps necessary to start your journey toward Self-Mastery and healing yourself. Congratulations and Wellness Warrior Salute.

HANIFF G7 a.k.a. Níff BIKō,
Wellness Warrior from the 7th SUNS Formation

TRUE SELF WITHIN

Man, Heal Thyself is a master key to self-healing and self-mastery. This text reflects not only Man's potential but also Man's destiny. It imparts confidence, understanding, wisdom, and discipline, helping Men remember and rediscover the true self within. Since reading this book and implementing its practices, I've found greater clarity of purpose, a deepened understanding of self, and a more profound ability to lead myself and my family. The guidance and practices provided in this book and the Man Heal Thyself program have helped me release trauma and blockages from my body and heart and have sharpened me mentally. Man Heal Thyself is a call and an answer to awaken.

Our love & gratitude,
Wellness Warrior Londrelle
Eternal Sunshine, LLC

THANK YOU

**My testimonial truly endorses the love, support, impeccable timing, and presence of Queen Afua, SupaNova Slom, Halleluyah Walcott, and all of the great Wellness Warriors and Sacred Women who I feel honored to call Brothers and SiStars, in the highest honor. I continue to build upon the amazing teachings and information shared. I also endorse their holistic products as some of the best in the market!!!

WW Bjm@studiobjm.com
ByronJohnMoore |studiobjm™
Visual and Performing Arts|
Holistic Wellness Practitioner|

WHO BETTER THAN US?

Man Heal Thyself, what a transformative experience. I challenge all men—small, tall, black, white, crippled, or crazy—to take this journey. Who better than you? What time is better than now to get acquainted with your highest and wisest self? It's an invaluable experience and you'll form a brotherhood that will last a lifetime. Self-love, Self-mastery, Self-discovery. Take the leap; your body is willing, but the mind and spirit need some healing. Answer the call!! See you on the front line!!

Wellness Warrior Salute!! Ru! Ru! Ru!
Wellness Warrior~Saleem Pasha

A SAFE SPACE

I am honored to share my experience with the Man Heal Thyself: Rites of Passage Program. Before entering this journey, I felt disconnected from my true self, lacking a sense of direction and purpose. Like many men, I was carrying emotional baggage and unresolved pain that I had buried deep within, believing that I could push through life without confronting it. But deep down, I knew I needed a transformation. The Man Heal Thyself rites of passage offered me a safe space and structure to go through a process that was not only empowering but deeply healing. From the very first moment, I felt welcomed and understood. The calls provided an environment where vulnerability was not only accepted but encouraged. This was the first time I had ever truly felt safe enough to confront my fears, my insecurities, and the unhealed wounds I had been carrying for years.

The physical, emotional, and spiritual exercises were intense, but they were exactly what I needed to face the parts of myself that I had been avoiding. Each step of the journey was thoughtfully designed to challenge me in different ways, helping me to reconnect with my own strength, my ancestral roots, and the balance of divine masculinity/femininity that lies within every man. The rituals, the group sharing, and the solo time for reflection all allowed me to peel back the layers of conditioning I had been living under and embrace the God I was meant to be.

What was most powerful for me was the deep sense of brotherhood that emerged throughout the process. The men I was with were not strangers—they were brothers who were walking a similar path. We shared our stories, held space for one another, and encouraged each other to heal. I felt a level of support and camaraderie that I had never experienced before. There was no judgment, only compassion, and it was through that collective healing that I was able to begin healing myself.

By the end of the rites, I walked away with a renewed sense of purpose, inner peace, and a deeper connection to my authentic self. I had faced the shadows of my past and emerged stronger, more grounded, and more aligned with my true essence. The Man Heal Thyself program didn't just teach me how to heal; it showed me that healing is a lifelong journey, and I now have the tools to continue that journey with strength, clarity, and confidence.

If you are a man who is ready to step into your full power and heal the wounds of your past, I wholeheartedly recommend this program. It is a transformative experience that will leave you forever changed.

Much Thanks and Love go out to Queen Afua, Halleluyah, and SupaNova for creating and facilitating such Divine Rites of Passage.

—Wellness Warrior King Kaos Da God
KING OF THE KONKRETE JUNGLE!

ASCEND TO YOUR HIGHER SELF

Wellness Warrior Salute. This is Brother (7god) tapping in from formation number 5, aka the fist.

My rites of passage experience was beautiful, ugly, challenging, and liberating, all at the same time. Coming into my 30th solar return, my family asked me what I desired. My only reply was to become a better version of myself. I am in full gratitude for the Wellness Warrior Rites of Passage program.

I learned so many things about myself, from strength to weaknesses, as well as tools needed to help me become my optimal self.

I recommend this to any man who is looking to heal, build, and ascend to their higher self; this rites of passage is a must for you. From the wellness baths, to the extensive knowledge of herbs, to the beautiful accountability from righteous brotherhood, there are so many things about being a man I didn't know until I took this program. God willing, if you are reading this you are on the righteous path. So, with that being said, it's time for you to . . .

Ase.

MAY I BE STRONG

Arrange for me the way. May I renew myself. May I be strong. This mantra set the tone for my wellness journey with my brothers, the 7th Suns. It was one of the darkest times in my life, leading me to reach out to SupaNova Slom, the Commander in Health. Within a single year, I lost my dad, my career of 22 years, and my fiancée. Amidst this storm, however, came the greatest gift I could ever receive—my son was born. A bittersweet time, indeed.

I sank into a deep depression, filled with anger, resentment, and a hollow hatred for life. Every day, I felt like I wanted to disappear. My family relationships suffered, I distanced myself from friends, and my eating and fitness habits fell apart. Shame, guilt, and frustration weighed heavily on me. It was my best friend, Tobi, who saved me from this ocean of despair, encouraging me to seek help. I cried, I yelled, and I took on all the blame, whether or not it was in my control.

Then, I knew it was time. I reached out to SupaNova, and he responded immediately. The program began in two weeks, and I joined without hesitation. This was the best decision of my life. Becoming a Wellness Warrior hasn't made life easy—it has made me more focused and stronger in my resolve. Now I am better equipped to handle life's challenges. I am a Wellness Warrior, every hour of every day. When dark times come, I command a life of abundance, affirming that when the road gets rough, I will remain unbothered. The shadow fades within 72 hours because I am anchored in light.

Wellness Warrior Salute,
James Rogers AKA Solar Allah
Son of Light and Righteousness
Health and Wellness Coach in DC

CONTINUED HEALING

Wellness Warrior Salute, Brothers!

If you are reading this testimony, it means that in this moment you have chosen to affirm yourself by looking in the mirror at your divine reflection, for we are all connected, and through our stories we gather strength, endurance, and self-determination. I am the husband of a Sacred Woman and the Father of three beautiful Daughters. When I went through the MHTS process in the 3rd formation, I was on the verge of a divorce and the destruction of my family. Our finances were in bankruptcy, and to compound these issues we were in the midst of a deadly pandemic.

Through the MHTS program I learned vital wellness practices such as spiritual baths, herbal teas, and speaking powerful words over myself before each sunrise. I would love to be able to tell you that things got easier after our ascension, but they did not. The details of my life were exactly where I left them when I began the process. The only difference was the investment I made in myself and gaining the tools that I applied consistently to improve my situation. I still got Covid-19, but I had learned how to use herbs to heal myself and recover.

I still struggled in my marriage, but I had learned how to journal and how to be accountable to myself so that I was making the most of my time between therapy sessions. However, a lesson that I had to learn the hard way is that healing myself is a very different process from healing a broken relationship. I had to learn that forgiving myself for the things I had done to myself and others is very different from obtaining forgiveness and reconciliation from the Woman I hurt.

My Wife and I were separated for a year and were at the point of meeting with lawyers and signing paperwork, but I was persistent in my altar work, and so was She. Even though we had all but agreed to go our separate ways, we were both dedicated to ensuring our family found safe harbor. What we did not realize at first was that this did not just include the children, but also each other. It was during this process that I learned what it meant to love someone unconditionally, regardless of outcome, and without sacrificing my own boundaries. To be the Lover Man of Harmony, I had to learn how to let go and hold on at the same time.

Today, my Wife and I are stronger than ever. We are celebrating 15-plus years of marriage, but it feels like this is year one—the second time. I went through the MHTS process a second time in the 8th formation. I am still not where I want to be, but I am making progress. I am in the process of healing my family and healing my bloodline. I am in the process of healing my body and healing my finances. I am in the process of my progress and my growth increases exponentially each day.

May you progress in your daily work, Brothers. Wellness Warrior Salute.

Anthony "Fatalprose" Miller

SUPPORTIVE SACRED WOMEN

Included here are excerpts from some of the Wellness Warriors' reflections, as well as comments from Supportive Sacred Women, some of the wives of Wellness Warriors.

ONE MAN'S JOURNEY

The MHT Wellness Warrior Rites of Passage Program was truly life changing for me. The tools that I gained along with the knowledge of applying them is invaluable. I was able to awaken parts of myself that I had either forgotten or believed were out of my reach. I had ignored them, and soon discovered I was not alone in this behavior.

As Program Director I had the unique opportunity to connect with other brothers and further strengthen our bonds. Faced with challenges, I have a multitude of allies in the daily fight for wellness. I noticed that I began to see myself differently, speak differently, and most importantly think differently. For the very first time I was able to fully accept my Victorious glory. However, the work is not done. The work has just begun, and this program has given me the inside track to achieving my optimal wellness.

Along with SupaNova, I had the ultimate honor of watching the men discover their own power while reestablishing their inner value. Men from different backgrounds, generations, and locations transformed in front of my eyes. That makes MHTWW Rites of Passage Program worth every bit of the work. I am excited because I know we are just beginning. The World of Wellness is . . . growing. Ascended Wellness Warriors are walking in their truth. They are lighting the way for their loved ones, for their communities, and for the world to see.

To the Queens, I give the utmost gratitude for seeing something in me that I did not see in myself and for entrusting me with this most powerful purpose. Wellness Warrior Salute!

Wellness Warrior Halleluyah Walcott
MHT Program Director
Los Angeles, California

FOREVER A WELLNESS WARRIOR

Man Heal Thyself is a brotherhood of Wellness Warriors that contributes to your success, while keeping you aligned on your climb to optimal wellness. Ascending through this program will give you all the tools and keys for your mind, body, and spirit to heal thyself. There is no judgment, just tough love, because it is your responsibility to hold to your commitment.

Man Heal Thyself is for every man in search of healing thyself, their children, ancestors, loved ones, and community. Going through MHT changed my perspective on life. I made a complete 360° from what I rise up doing, to what I don't do before I rest, including what I think and how I process my thoughts, emotions, words, and actions. You will forever have Wellness Warriors at the ready for you after becoming one. Ase, Ase, Ase, Ase-O!

Zakai Israel Gillman
New York, New York

HEALING MY RELATIONSHIP TRAUMA

The 2020 Man Heal Thyself Wellness Warrior Rites of Passage Program was a phenomenal program to be a part of. It was an honor to take part in Queen Afua's program and to read her book *Man, Heal Thyself*. I was able to transform into my wellness journey of healing physically, mentally, and spiritually. The program helped me to release and heal some relationship trauma that I had been holding and be at peace with some past bad decisions in my life. I was reminded that I was important and that I needed to take care of myself before I could possibly take care of someone else. I interacted with some incredible brothers. As we built bonds, we reached out to help one another without judgment. I learned what types of herbs could heal my body and was taught a path to optimal wellness which I'm grateful for. Thank you, Queen Afua!

Mark "Cool Breeze" Williams
Police Officer with the Hempstead Police Department
Long Island, New York

SUBLIME TRANSFORMATION

I am SWP Trae Nfr Williams, wife of WW Mark "Cool Breeze" Williams and mother of three. In 2017 my husband and sons attended a two-part Rites of Passage Ascension Ceremony (Sacred Woman and Man Heal Thyself). Mark is and has always been the "strong, silent" type. Educated, well-spoken, and not easily persuaded. As the women made their presentations, I noticed my husband occasionally glancing up and down at his cell phone. However, during the men's presentations, I noticed my King's eyes stayed glued with unwavering attention.

Over the next three years, my Mark joined the journey . . . in his own time and in his own way. He attended Ascension Ceremonies, prepared Green Life Formula, and even supported Queen Afua as stagehand for several presentations. Queen kept saying, "Man Heal Thyself Mark, hold on. . . . the men's rites program is coming back . . ." Mark replied "Ok, Queen."

By April 2020, Mark asked me about healing stones and fabric for his altar. If I so much as straightened a stone that seemed crooked to me, he would notice and ask, "You've been on my altar?" (Laugh) I was amazed to witness what was taking place in our home and in Mark during his twelve Wellness Warrior weeks. It continues . . . my husband and I have co-founded In The Balance of Love, a holistic healing consultation and referral service.

The Unity in the Body scripture passage (I remember it from my childhood) sums up what I have in My Beloved Husband. Ephesians 4:16: "From Him the whole body, fitted and held together by every supporting ligament, grows and builds itself up in love through the work of each individual part." The Man Heal Thyself experience . . . truly a magnificent blessing . . . Tua NTR. Yours in Wellness.

Trae Nfr Muima Maat
Licensed Property & Casualty Risk Manager
Long Island, New York

TRANSFORMATION

> **"As iron sharpens iron, so one man sharpens another."**
> **Proverbs 21:17**

This verse holds true only after the men are given divine instruction. These instructions were repeated to us by our Sacred Queen Afua. Tua NTR to Queen Afua for pouring the Divine instructions from the Source on High into SupaNova Slom, Ali The Great, and Halleluyah Walcott, so that they can sharpen others. Tua NTR to our brothers who embraced their assignments . . . Tua NTR to those given life to assist with this charge. Tua NTR.

We experienced many life-changing instructions with the goal to make good men into better men. Exercises focused on the effects of our thinking and behavior. Previously we had constantly fallen backwards into toxic ways. This program gives us instructions for becoming wholesome men. Although we were from different environments, educational backgrounds, theologies, and financial statuses, we each saw our own story in our brothers' stories. We had one thing in common: We all needed healing. The most powerful thing was that there were no judgments.

We released the blockages we've been holding inside. Despite virtual participation, we "felt" our brothers' arms around us in comfort and protection. Their words were soothing and firm. Halleluyah opens and closes the way. What happens in between those two points in time? HMMMM . . . Never a dull moment . . .

MHT Wellness Warrior has given us the formula to Optimal Wellness. We received a regimen to keep our spirit in harmony with the tone of the OMniverse. We received tools to maintain a balanced state of mind. We received remedies to keep our body in optimal health. During those twelve weeks we each reclaimed Me, Myself, and I. We were becoming Disease-Free, Drama-Free, Drug-Free, and Debt-Free . . . plus becoming two belt sizes smaller.

LOL. I transformed from the inside of me to outward. I'm the son of Esther and Sydney; Father of Shayaa, Shelomoh, Shuaib, Yasmin, Temu, and AseT. I continue my wellness journey as student and teacher of Sciences, Culture, and Theology. I am a Wellness Warrior.

Every Nubian Nation, tribe, organization, and culture should implement Man Heal Thyself Wellness Warrior Rites of Passage into their ministry for the boys and men. "You are not ever too old to learn nor are you too young to teach. Give them life." Wellness Warrior "Aqua Man" Salute.

NeHisi aNKh SeKheM

Kemetic Yoga Instructor,
Kemetic Reiki 2 Practitioner, Entrepreneur
Earth (Augusta, Georgia)

WE ARE ACCOUNTABLE AT THE HIGHEST LEVEL

I am eternally grateful to be a Man Heal Thyself Wellness Warrior. All praises due to the Most High. I feel forever indebted to the Mothership of Queen Afua and Queen Esther. I know that their love for Men's Wellness led them to bestow the tutelage and guidance on SupaNova and Halleluyah in order that the Man Heal Thyself Rites of Passage would be manifested. Their collective vision, along with the contributions of many others, has been manifesting into Man Heal Thyself for decades.

When I became overwhelmed with the feeling of welcome, I knew I BELONGED HERE, in the ever-present Man Heal Thyself energy! I recognized that the way to reach optimal healing had already been made. I entered with notions that I had been living some areas of my life at optimal level. I soon learned that I could become stronger in ALL areas and truly become an Optimal Man of Wellness. The program material fed us spiritually, physically, and emotionally. The tools provided research-based practices to help ensure success. This program is the Truth! We were put on assignment to hold each other accountable at the highest level. As a military veteran, I know firsthand that there is no mission that is impossible for a fraternity or family acting in one accord. Man Heal Thyself makes Optimal Wellness possible for any and all Men who, as our esteemed Minister of Wellness SupaNova Slom charges, "Commit to the Commitment!" I am healed, I am healing, I am a healer. I am a Man Heal Thyself Wellness Warrior.

Kevin 'Addalesson' Graham

Founder of Head Full of STEAM LLC.

Systems Engineer

2021 BEYA Professional Achievement Nominee

Suffolk, Virginia

I AM A RENEWED HUSBAND, FATHER, SON & BROTHER

I acknowledge that I was raised with minimal tools. My parents did the best they could with what they had and showed me how to work . . . yet, honestly, we never got ahead. Early in life I adopted the idea of success being the ability to win in a system designed for my failure. I achieved a good bit of success in this American society, but at the cost of losing myself and turning into something unnatural.

Man Heal Thyself gave me information, tools, and a group of like-minded individuals I needed to complete work this intense. These blessings came at a time when we were advised to stay home by those who govern. Navigating the 12 rites of passage challenged and changed me. We were given Knowledge and Understanding, along with an accountability group to help guarantee transformation and success. But, most importantly, I learned that the buck stops with me.

I am a renewed Husband, Father, Son, and Brother. My son will have tools I never had, and his sons will have those tools. We will do uncomfortable work and surrender to the outcome. We will be Spiritually and physically fortified. I envision my future self and my relationships and my kid's kid's kids and our lives achieved through high vibrations and meaningful manifestations. I look forward to living and giving love and light. MHT taught me to Rise, Shine, Listen, Receive, and Activate. I give thanks, I give praise. Ase!

WW Hilton T. Ferguson II
Owner of "Fulltime Fitness"
High Point, North Carolina

MAN HEAL THYSELF: A DREAM COME TRUE

My family is of Nigerian descent. I enjoy photography, working out, reading, writing, podcasting, and spending time outside. My experience participating in the Man Heal Thyself Wellness Warrior Rites of Passage Program has been life-changing. I embarked on this journey not knowing the pain and emotional scars that I had accumulated over the years. Man Heal Thyself helped me locate and address them. The rituals and practices that were taught to me, I will utilize for the rest of my days. To join a community of like-minded gentlemen who want to live in holistic wellness has been a dream come true. I would recommend this rites of passage program to any man looking to better themselves for not only himself but for his family and loved ones.

Wale Orimogunje
IT Technical Support Specialist
Far Rockaway, Queens, New York

MY WHOLE LIFE BLOSSOMED

From NTR (The Creator) I have learned, the more you educate self, the more you understand where things come from . . . the more obvious things become. You begin to see lies everywhere. You have to know the truth. If I seek the truth, it will set me free. The day I met my Goodness Mother, Queen Afua, and my Brother the Supreme Being, SupaNova Slom, was the day my inner being blossomed. I began absorbing the brilliance of what living life in its entirety looks like in Ma'at.

As a wounded man, I had no conscious direction or sustainable purpose for living. My father wasn't around, so I looked up to the big boys and did what they did. The gift of my life was nothing special. I did foolish things which put my life in danger. Tomorrow wasn't promised and I wasn't looking for it. I overdid it with loud music which caused severe hearing damage. I messed up money and peoples' time. I didn't admit to or remember doing wrong things. My wife and I had been inseparable, but my behavior caused explosive arguments. I begged her to stay. I didn't want to die an old man in a cage. Sadly, I gave up and crawled into bed. The only doctor I knew was sleep. The day I had an aneurysm, someone called an ambulance to take me to the hospital. I survived, but there were repercussions because I never followed through with the treatments. My wife and kids tried to give me the peace I needed.

Queen Afua and SupaNova Slom are the epitome of life, in Ma'at. They are the prototype of love, peace, and light. Queen Afua nurtured me. Humbly, I accepted her invitation to attend the rites of passage class in March 2020. The first day of bootcamp the men received course details and goals. I met some of this galaxy's most brilliant Brothers. Reiki masters, authors, electricians, fitness experts, nuclear engineers, body builders. We challenged ourselves to endure the rigorous bootcamp of Optimal Wellness. Down-to-earth players, businessmen, herbalists, artists, producers, photographers, truck drivers, professors, scientists, KING MEN, ministers, philosophers, philanthropists, the culturally conscious . . . We became a Fraternity of Wellness Brothers. Weekly, we shared gifts of experiences and knowledge. We made a commitment to transform. We all came out of the mud we were in. Asé

As I began to ascend into the greatness I was born to be, my wife and I began to Yin & Yang, in Ma'at. The 12 chambers of Optimal Wellness groomed the Nefer Atun, vibrating these tones of testimony. I acquired Man Heal Thyself knowledge from the book and the rites program. I have intuitive clear vision. I have been equipped to move into the next dimensions of Wellness. I AM GLAD TO BE ALIVE.

I am Welmaker the Immortal Rey of LIFE. I am constantly ascending, consciously elevating toward Optimal Wellness. I am a Fearless Wellness Warrior! I am a Master Problem-Solver. I am the man that HEALS THYSELF. I was a union electrician. I was struggling to survive. I am a promoter of living an abundantly full life overflowing with greatness. I AM HEALING! ASÉ O HOTEP!

I am Welmaker the Immortal Rey of LIFE
Atlanta, Georgia

A VICTORIOUS JOURNEY

I began my journey on this planet 43 years ago. Little did I know of the power guiding me in opening my True Path and Divine Purpose. March 29th, 2020 was the first session in our Wellness Warriors Rites of Passage. That day is now forever engraved in My Being and My Heart. With every opening and closing of the Aritu Gateway sessions, there IS the life force power, sekhem, that rises in Me and my beloved brothers. As we journeyed through the Gateways (Aritu), I discovered more and more about the true inner and outer selves and cells.

The guidance of our beloved great Minister of Opening the Way, Hallelujah Walcott, and our beloved great Minister of Wellness, SupaNova Slom, has been and IS invaluable to me, my wife, and my two sons. Words could never express our Divine Gratitude for their energy, tones, and vibrations. This is more than wellness rites. This is the Unification of Our Divine and Sacred Ancestors moving through each of us. We are forever grateful! Through my alignment with my inner self, I have awakened, and therefore I can claim the restoration of Humanity! This has always been my Dream, Vision, and Goal! I see my Divine Purpose unfolding before me. I have Known this since my childhood days.

Throughout my journey, the mud of trials and tribulations had caused stagnation, amnesia, and forgetfulness. My Brothers reflect my Self and cells! Now, My Brothers, The Mothership, and my Highest most Optimal Self are ready to embark on the journey of Divine Natural! I am a Living Soul—sovereign, indigenous, and retained. A student teacher of the Master Teacher.

I am married to a Sacred Woman and I am a Blessed Father of Two Suns. Together WE ALL work in unison to unite as ONE. I am Giving Life to the service of others and the healing of Our People. I am Giving life to the service of others and the healing of Our People. MAN HEAL THYSELF!! I am a Wellness Warrior! WELLNESS WARRIOR SALUTE!! Ase!

AmSu SaHu RE
A Respiratory Therapist by Trade,
Entrepreneur, Budding Master Herbalist
Miami, Florida

CRAFTY NOT CRAZY, PURPOSEFUL NOT PUSHY

The awesome bonding and building of a spiritual, metaphysical, upfront, and in-your-face brotherhood with the goal of being a better MAN. Direct, empowering, insightful, uplifting, crafty not crazy, purposeful not pushy. The combination of the young, intelligent, committed, resourceful, talented leaders was planned from the love, care, and concern of some very insightful and unique people.

The Man Heal Thyself Rites of Passage was life-changing. It allowed me an opportunity to explore unknown parts of my life and purpose. At this point I was able to search and find meaningful, promising aspects of fulfilling my life vocation.

Shawn Thomas
IT Expert and Transportation Specialist
Trenton, New Jersey

HEALING LEADS TO RESTORATION

Witnessing my beloved's journey through the Man Heal Thyself Rites of passage was such a beautiful experience. His healing journey was literally the catalyst for the restoration of our relationship, as he introduced me to the "new him." I was extremely proud and honored to support him throughout his journey. His life has forever been changed, and so has our bond. This amazing program will reunite the "Black Family." Asé!

Sacred Woman Practitioner Ayanna Williams
(Wife of Wellness Warrior Shawn Thomas)
Artisan, Massage Therapist, Owner/Founder of
Aya Earth Wellness, LLC.
New Jersey

WELLNESS WARRIOR SALUTE

TO MY VICTORIOUS BROTHERS

I would like to Open the Way of this heartfelt missive by giving thanks to The One Most High and Our Sacred Ancestors. I am beyond grateful to Queen Afua for bringing Black Men together so we can achieve her vision of health and wellness and become the paramount reality for ourselves and our families. It has been an honor and a blessing to have been a member of the first class of Wellness Warriors.

I have learned so many things from each and every one of my Brothers. This Collective of Black Genius has forged a better understanding of unity and kinship within my mind, spirit, and physical well-being. Our leadership Halleluyah and Supa-Nova Slom's complementary style of bringing forth the Black-Print and the essential reawakening of our Alpha Male-selves cannot truly be put into words other than, Give Thanks, Super Men! Ase!

Enen Kes Maa
Real Estate
Brooklyn, New York

IT'S ALL UP TO YOU

This journey has been a long one for my husband. He was an arrogant womanizer mister ("I think I know everything, I don't care about anyone, not even my children . . .") until he realized he had lost everything . . . me included. I had had enough, and so had our children. We completely turned our backs on him. He was lost and alone and desperate for some type of healing. It started with me first. So, I joined the Sacred Woman rites of passage, and so did our two daughters, Sacred Woman T'Annu Nepheara and Sacred Woman Ariana Frazier.

My husband saw the shift that we all had made without him. Still he needed to do some self-care. This time he took the advice from me and Queen Afua to take the Man Heal Thyself program. At first he was very resistant. He didn't want to listen to his instructors. He kept saying, "They can't help me." So, I told him, "That's fine, you know everything, and you quit. But know this: We won't be waiting around for you this time. IT'S ALL UP TO YOU."

Long story short, he started taking his journey seriously. He started eating better, getting up in the mornings, meditating, and doing his altar work. He started speaking to the children better and treating me better. The shift for me was when the girls said, "Daddy is different." They started listening to him. I was like, "Wow, ok, I see you!" The transformation was incredible. Yes, he did some back-sliding into his old ways. I overstand that we are not perfect. We are HUMAN. I've learned to stay silent. I let him go through what is bothering him until he is ready to talk. After that, he gets his mind right . . . lol. EVERY MAN SHOULD TAKE THE MAN HEAL THYSELF PROGRAM.

SW, SWP, WYDP, EGP & MUT Snefer Ausaraqa.
Wife of Wellness Warrior Enen Kes Maa (Keith Frazier)

HEAL OUR TRAUMA

Man Heal Thyself program had a subtle but powerful impact on my life. The program came at the perfect time. During the era of Covid-19, it was extremely beneficial to be reminded to stay committed to our commitment. We have to pour into ourselves so that we can pour into the ones we love. I was also able to heal past traumas of abandonment and misguided leadership and see them from a healed and healthy perspective. The subtle things that I learned will always stay with me on my journey, and I am grateful to have shared those moments with the brothers of the Man Heal Thyself fraternity. Queen Afua wanted me to be a part of this program for a long time. It is truly an honor to have fulfilled that vision.

Mentchu Ma'at
Entrepreneur
Brooklyn, New York

EMERALD GREEN HOLISTIC PRACTITIONERS

Emerald Green Holistic Practitioners have studied and are certified in the principles and practices of a holistic lifestyle.

Emerald Green Holistic Practitioners are Wellness Warriors because they are ready to defend the wellness of their clients/students.

SAVED MY LIFE

Peace and blessings to all of my wellness warrior brothers. My name is De'Arcy BA-RA, and Man Heal Thyself has changed my life. I come from a family of very strong Queens. My grandmother and mother raised me, so I know the power of a woman and the healing that takes place when there is no resistance.

I once ate pork, beef, junk food, fast food, microwaved food, EVERY DAY! My mother had to work two jobs, so I had to survive the best way I knew how. I read Queen Afua's Heal Thyself, and it changed my life. After witnessing my grandmother's illness, my mother's struggle, and my own sister's womb being taken right in front of me—all relating to an unhealthy lifestyle, I had to learn and quickly! As my sister screamed for a ride to the hospital every month, and my grandmother could not leave her bed, I said, "THAT'S IT! NO MORE!! I will awaken the healer within and Heal Thyself, and my Queens."

Queen Afua saved my life. I am now an Emerald Green Holistic Practitioner and a strict vegan. My family understands that liberation comes through purification. Man Heal Thyself is my guide, my sword, my protection.

De'Arcy BA-RA
Journalist/Artist

GRATITUDE FOR HEALING

Through my study as an Emerald Green Holistic Practitioner, I've become conscious that I am a seer—I see a lot of life much clearer. I accept that I am a healer. But before I guide others to Wellness I had to be sure that my health was intact. I had to start healing the "Man in the Mirror." I had to Heal Thyself to become a temple, clean and pure. I drink and eat foods that are green and raw. With every sip and bite, I add years to my life. I am Emerald Green straight to the heart. I will not part from the Emerald Green life. I'm not a flexitarian, vegan, or vegetarian. I'm a straight up Emerald Green Chlorophyllin.

I give thanks and praise to the Most High and the ancestors. I give thanks and praise to my mother for being the vessel through which I returned. She taught me the importance of a holistic lifestyle, how to be truly spiritual and introduced the teachings of Queen Afua to my brother and sister and me. I give thanks and praise to my wife and children for travelling with me on this wellness journey. I give thanks and praise to Queen Afua for your teachings and guidance and also bestowing upon me the title of Emerald Green Holistic Practitioner and "Supa-Man." May the Most High continue to use you as a vessel for healing. We've only just begun. Now the real work comes, because we Wellness Warriors have a mission to fulfill. Queen Afua, you are the Queen of Green. Hotep.

Brother Heru Jamal
Security, Harlem Hospital

I WILL NOT DIE

I will not die while I am living, numbing myself,
  burying the pain.
I will fully live a life of healing.
I will not die. I will live, while living.

I will not die from violence or a tragic accident.
I will not die because I didn't eat right.
I will not die from living a toxic life.
I will not die from any unhealthy reason.
I will not die from not fasting every new season.
I will not die because my body is purified and my
healthy glow shows it.
I will not die because my body is the temple that
holds my spirit.
I will not die because I'm one with the most high
and I know it.
I will not die because my spirit is immortal.
I will not die because my soul travels back and
forth through the heavenly portals.
I will not die because I've learned my life lessons.
I will live in the spiritual,
So when the time comes that I transcend my
physical,
I will not die.
These are simple truths that I can't deny.
These are the reasons
I will not die.

By Heru Jamal

QUEEN AFUA'S RESPONSE TO "I WILL NOT DIE"

As man grows in age, parts of the body will break down if they have not been protected by a wellness lifestyle. Disease mounts: Body systems shut down and body parts are cut away while the man is still alive. Men who smoke, drink, snort and shoot up drugs, consume toxic foods, and constantly have non-love-giving sexual experiences are inviting death sooner rather than later.

The early signs of death are arthritis, diabetes, prostate

cancer, Alzheimer's, depression, and low libido. A toxic lifestyle eats away at the body, mind, and soul. Man Heal Thyself and live fully. Walk strong in spirit and enjoy loving yourself. Learn your lessons and forgive your past. Thank your parents for carrying you to full term. DO NOT die while living. Instead, bond with your brothers in Wellness. Open your heart, offer gratitude out loud, form circles of healing. Spread the love. But most importantly, DO NOT die while living. Affirm daily, "I Will Not Die. I Will Live."

Queen Afua

WITNESSES TO WELLNESS

These Witnesses to Wellness have studied and applied the Man Heal Thyself principles into their own lives for many years. Their experience qualifies these witnesses to testify to the benefits of living a Man Heal Thyself lifestyle.

I JUST WANNA TESTIFY

When I first met Queen Afua, I knew she would take a part in changing my life. She spoke life and promoted life. SO MANY of us want to live long, yet we intake the souls of dead animals when we eat their flesh. So many are so quick to say, "I can't give up my pork, beef, and chicken." But they don't realize that eating those things is what cuts our lives short. Queen Afua's third book, *The City of Wellness: Restoring Your Health Through the Seven Kitchens of Consciousness*, is where I was introduced to the deadly impact of the "Corporate Kitchen" and what to do to recover from the diseases one can get by eating in a bad way. Queen Afua made me aware that I could heal myself. I salute the Queen because she was the first to talk to me about life with the solution being life. N.O.R.E follows Queen, SO SHOULD YOU!

Noreaga
Hip-Hop Artist

FROM DEATH TO REJUVENATION

My mother passed away when I was 8 years old. As a result, I suffered great losses throughout my life. I've worked on my recovery in different programs. I didn't understand how my body worked until I found Man Heal Thyself. First, I am grateful to have the blessing of successfully completing attendance for natural healing in the Man Heal Thyself Program.

Queen Afua helped me to restore my life. I didn't understand the scroll and the teachings as a daily practice until she taught me. This is why I found the Man Heal Thyself 28-Day Detoxification Program so beneficial. Queen Afua's weekly guidance, her creation of the Man Heal Thyself Scrolls, The City of Wellness Nutrition Kitchen Laboratory Chart, and the Liberation Diet Pyramids of Wellness were the tools I used for changing eating habits. With Queen Afua's formulas, I achieved control of my acute diabetes. At my age, 73, I'm much more alive than I was before. The spiritual touching that I needed occurs when Queen Afua speaks. I didn't know how to change my life or my eating habits. I had no help. I knew I was detoxified after two weeks of taking Queen Afua's formulas and living the Man Heal Thyself natural lifestyle. All foul eliminations ceased, there was no more constipation, body odor, bad back, or bad eyesight. It was ALL GONE! I can see the road and read the signs while driving at night. I am beginning the reversal of erectile dysfunction. I now sleep through the night without getting up to urinate every two hours as I was previously required to do. Because I have had great improvements in my mental state, I am registering to re-enter the practice of law. I recommend to all the men that you attend the next Man Heal Thyself training. Do not miss this opportunity to rejuvenate and refresh your body, spirit, and mind. I send love to you on your journey to a healthier lifestyle.

Kenneth Hagood, Esq.

THE OPENING OF THE WAY

The first day that I came under the direct personal influence of Queen Afua and her Heal Thyself: Green Road Map to Optimal Wellness Program happened in July 2011. I had already attended Queen Afua's City of Wellness Seminars twice at the National Black Theatre in Harlem. Without any doubt, Queen Afua's program has been the "Opening of the Way" for my personal healing.

Economic, social, political, intellectual, and spiritual oppression have ruled over my family for generations. We consumed unhealthy food and drank daily for many years. We grew up in the inner city of New York as a part of the working poor. We did not know why or how our profound social illnesses came about. Before the teachings of the Honorable Elijah Muhammad, author of the classic book *How to Eat to Live*, no one ever taught us how food made our very own deep-rooted illnesses, wickedness, and sickness permanent.

Queen Afua's Heal Thyself: Green Road Map to Optimal Wellness Program and the Man Heal Thyself Wellness Program have raised my health consciousness to a higher level. I started applying her recommended approach to my daily menu. I realized that I am in the process of making a lifestyle transformation which will last for the rest of my life. My wife and I have begun the process of transforming our kitchen into a Healing Kitchen Laboratory. Queen Afua has created a chart entitled The Liberation Diet Pyramids of Wellness which outline this process.

Our family is beginning to enjoy the benefits of changing our lifestyle and healing ourselves and reaching for our optimal wellness.

Hannibal Ahmed
Historian Researcher

HOLISTIC WELLNESS LUMINARIES SPEAK

These Witnesses to Wellness are outstanding practitioners in their fields of discipline. They have each incorporated the Man Heal Thyself principles in their teachings for many years.

WHAT IS TIME? WHAT TIME IS IT?

LLoyd Strayhorn

As an AstroNumerologist, time means everything to me. First of all, time is of the essence! Now, you can take your sweet time if you want to, but time moves with precision and waits for no one. Time is a measure of things. Time is a guide of how long one has to do things and how much gets done. Imagine, for example, telling a woman baking bread in the oven that she can come back to check on it "anytime" she wishes, let's say, next week or next month? With that miscalculation of the time needed to do the task it would be a wonder if she came back in a week and still had an oven left in the kitchen, much less the bread.

But we do not have to imagine appropriate or inappropriate uses of time. We can and must focus on what time it is now. It is time to get things done in a quick and orderly manner. Most importantly, it is time that every man—young and old—pick up a copy of Queen Afua's amazing book, *Man, Heal Thyself: Journey to Optimal Wellness.* It is time that we men act on the truth and the power to be found within the pages of this book. Men, we must begin the process of moving from "Wounded Man to Supreme Man of Optimal Wellness."

It has always been a given that Queen Afua's role, among

many, is to empower women, especially with regard to their health. That comes as no surprise if you've ever had the pleasure of meeting this wonder spirit. Her smile is like the sun, the symbol of her zodiac sign, Leo. More importantly, being around her aura or presence is healing in itself. When you can't help but return a smile, you end up listening to what she is talking about. And, many have been listening. Over the years I have personally observed how the health of clients of mine had improved once they began eating naturally and organically as Queen suggests. Now, men, it is time for us to begin to pay attention to our healing. As you get into this jewel of a book, it's obvious that Queen Afua is very aware of the male species and our way of thinking, acting, and Being. Queen Afua's *Man, Heal Thyself: Journey to Optimal Wellness* provides checklists to get us up to speed and keep us on track. Step-by-step, she guides us to raise our awareness, heighten our consciousness, and understand the true role healthy living habits play on our state of being.

What is required of us men is to own up to the myths and misplaced motives we have about ourselves and our relationships. It is time to take responsibility for our behavior, which eventually has an impact not only on our lives but also on the women and children in our lives. *Man, Heal Thyself* should be shared with the younger generation to guide them to become better individuals. To delay reading this book or to delay beginning the processes outlined in this book would be unwise. The last thing we need to do is waste our precious time. Men, we need to be where we men need to be; and we need to get on time about it. The value of reading and working through this guide to personal growth and development is priceless. Learning to actually transform yourself and your life in ways that you haven't experienced in years, or maybe ever, should be enough to motivate any man. Wow . . . just the thought of it staggers the imagination!

IT IS TIME!

World Renowned Astro-Numerologist and Bestselling Author
Numbers and You: A Numerology Guide for Everyday Living
Lloyd's Numbers and You Workbook:
A Basic Guide to Numerology
https://www.lloyd-strayhorn.com/

THE CALL OF MAN HEAL THYSELF

Baba Wanique Khemi~Tehuti Shabazz

MAN HEAL THYSELF WELLNESS WARRIOR! What a perfect affirmation for the closing of the cycle of patriarchal rule and toxic male dominance. The commencement of **history, August 13, 3113** BC *(13.0.0.0 Long Count)* to the end date of the Olmec-Mayan Great Cycle **12-21-12. (A significant and synchronistic Gregorian date of "August 13" is also the Solar Return and incarnation date for SW High Priestess Queen Afua**) This *"Closing of the Cycle"* was a cosmic event, a rare passage in the eon; the impossibly immense cycle containing all the other cycles was itself but a fractal of a divine thought-moment. The smallest cycle closing then is the Great Cycle of **history**, a span of **5,125** years from **Babylon** to **Baghdad.**

The recent "Great Jupiter-Saturn Conjunction" of **12-21-20** placed us on the steady alignment trajectory of relevant significance insofar as relating to the Harmonic Convergence of Greg **12-21-12,** where major cycles converged into that one calendrical moment—shifting the trajectory of energy and ushering in the close of Babylonian rule and influence through its macro & micro (calendar/clock) programming devices, respectively. JUPITER & SATURN have always had a great influence on our planet and thereby our 3rd & 4th dimensional activities. This conjunction will certainly intensify what many are already experiencing, as the "great" shift continues to clear our toxic psyche for an expanded awareness and higher consciousness, particularly in these overtly turbulent times of biological & psychological germ warfare.

This reminder is, of course, based on the re**membering** of Ausar's 14 pieces that were scattered across the planet. It is only through the prophetic call of a Sacred Wombman that amending of the severed dismembered pieces can be gathered and reconnected. The amnesiac virus that has permeated this planet we call Earth has placed us, *men & women,* at odds with each other and divided against ourselves. The left & right sides of the human anatomy are screaming for reunification and a return to wholeness, a return to the oneness of ourselves granted to us by our parents (pair-entities).

Our disconnect from and discontent with our parents are the primary sources of maladies and dis-ease in our sacred temples simply because biologically, we are their bodies joined together by sharing the 46 chromosomes that the sperm (23) and the egg (23) culminate in harmony to be. Our adult resentments and failed expectations of our initial childhood stages of development are the diagnostic cause of our chronic illness. Until we come to grips and "make peace with our parents," all our illness will be unsustainable and incurable by the chemistry of judgment and unforgiveness. The temporary relief from the ancient bush women remedies and wellness potions provided by Mother Queen won't give us full rehabilitation to the recidivism of "cell" degeneration.

The imbalance is seen in our physiological structure. The left brain is directly responsible for controlling our anatomy's right body function. The Indigenous Hopis call this control metaphorically on a world level "the triumph of the clever side, the right side of the body with no heart." Thus, we are resorting to data and information overload as the basis for sound intuitive telepathic knowing, better known as "Mother wit."

This explains the imbalance that we have lived under, with never-ending wars and the apocalyptic overt and covert ecological destruction of the biosphere of Mother Earth. This is also demonstrated in the repression, suppression, and oppression of women, i.e., the right brain and the left side. It is further played out in the erroneous illusion that the Earth as Mother is apart from the glory and nirvana of the "Heavens" and thereby separate from the larger galaxy that we look "up" to and aspire to reach. Earth is an integral planetary body of the "milky way" celestial bodies, 3rd in succession to the Sun; it is, in fact, also residing in the "Heavens."

With the end of this cycle, the intent is to return to all life's inclusiveness in which the feminine principle personifies. With all the programming spells that have been cast through internet social media, television programs, inaccurate, ineffective, and unsubstantiated educational institutions, the most notable spell is the *"spell"* of words. It is clear that within the dialect of the "English" language, the inclusiveness of gender is defined by s**he**, **her**, wo**man**, fe**male**, etc. The exclusion is obvious in the spell of "he," "man," "male," and so on. The third-dimensional biological fact that all men and women come through women is cause for pause and appreciation for her gender-specific job description—a divine reproductive act of creation as GOD. The mere physiological fact that *all* humans have mended umbilical cords (*aka* lifelines) gives credence to the female body's physical superiority. Does this irrefutable fact diminish or demoralize the importance of men? Absolutely not; it merely places us back in orbit with the synergy and the cause for physiologic presence. It also takes us to the germinating preparation for life within the cycles of 13 moons, 28 "days," which is in direct contradiction to the 12-month Gregorian calendar, which has nothing to do with the annual biological rhythm of the human species in harmony with the biosphere.

We have been programmed to "Artificial Intelligence" (AI) via machines (clock and watches) to gauge our navigation and our intrinsic value and worth a la the axiom "Time is Money." A clock does not measure time; it measures increments of space, which, projected as increments of time, are valorized into monetary units. Money is a function of false time, 12:60 (12 months 60 minutes). True-time is from the biosphere. Thirteen moons, 28 days is the biosphere's measure of the annual human biological rhythm of 28 days. Twenty-eight days 13 times a year is the human female *men*struation cycle. She is the epitome of creation; she *man*ifests all sentient beings. Everything is born of a woman. To kill a woman, to harm a child, is to destroy the potential of any biological future; this is the 12:60 way, the way of man-driven and instigated war. Men HIStorically perpetuate death, while women eternally perpetuate life. We take for granted that the calendar is the function of governance for society; it is the basis for all control and dominance.

MAN HEAL THYSELF WELLNESS WARRIOR is a call to release ourselves from this control and dominance in order to reclaim our autonomy. In order for us to be released from under the Vatican's colonial spell. It is the one unchallenged and non-protected instrument of the imperialist. Virtually all governments, the Vatican included, along with banking institutions worldwide, operate by the 12-month Gregorian calendar.

This calendar denies and covers up the true annual human biological cycle conserved in the body of women. These pertinent questions further exasperate the patriarchal rule: Why are virtually all government leaders men? Why is it that men make war? Why is it that men run all the banks?

Why are only men allowed to be priests in the Catholic Church? If you do the math, you can unlock the Gregorian calendar's spell by merely giving all months a sequence of 28 days and counting the remaining balance.

The call by Sacred Woman Queen Afua for **MAN HEAL THYSELF WELLNESS WARRIOR** is so timely. It is a trumpet sounding to clean up the mess that our physical existence reeks of. Through the work of Natural Time, I define this MESS as an acronym for the intangible Mental, Emotional, Spiritual & Soul issues calcified as blockages in our physical tissues. The idea that men can continue to perpetuate false dominance and superiority to women is seen in all aspects of our society. As men, we have much to account for in our behavior as a "privileged" & "entitled" displaced character in a world run and operated by the systemic practices of Euro-Western thought just by virtue of the male avatar we were born into. Our cultural distortion has made us replicas of the demoralizing and destabilizing society that diminishes the high value of women, and we have to now commit to being focused and more spiritually grounded and more committed to our life-purpose.

The call of **MAN HEAL THYSELF WELLNESS WARRIOR** is a resounding call for support, a call for accountability and responsibility. This is demonstrated in the Olmec-Mayan Prophecy of 2012, where Time's Special Witness, **Pacal Votan**, the Mayan Prophet's tomb was discovered on **Greg-June 15, 1952,** deep within the Pyramid of The Inscriptions. The return of the feminine is illustrated in the hieroglyphs within the Pyramids of Palenque Mexico and revealed to us through the work of Jose Arguelles-Valum Votan: The Closer of the Cycle, in this quote from **Living through the Closing of the Cycle—A Survival Guide for the Road to 2012:**

> "Until the discovery of the tomb of the **Red Queen** on **Greg-June 1, 1994,** Pacal's tomb was considered

> unique, but the tomb of the **Red** Queen (so-called because her otherwise jade bedecked corpse was covered with cinnabar) in the adjacent Temple XIII (13), was a further clue. Identical to that of Pascal, the tomb of the **Red Queen** also featured a jade mask and a speaking tube. The only difference between the two tombs is that the tomb of Pacal Votan is laden with inscriptions, while that of the Red Queen has none. These two tombs are those of inter-dimensional travelers, intentionally placed to be a sign for us in the end times. Pascal's inscribed tomb details points of passage from previous world systems. The Red Queen's tomb represents the future yet to be inscribed. That she, too, wore a jade mask—the sign of having acquired a true face or being enlightened—showed that the Red Queen was the spiritual heir of the Great Pascal.
>
> We can all be on the 2013 red road of feminine resurrection after the long-awaited end-cycle of the black road-2012."

(It is this prophetic revelation that lends to the spiritual significance and divine importance of the healing work of SW Queen Afua—White Overtone Wind Kin 122.)

The **300**-year period of the infamous "**1712** Willie Lynch Papers" has us at the crossroads, and it is leading us to restore the **LAWS of MA'AT** commensurate to the **LAW of TIME** at the culminating threshold of **2012**. These immutable laws give us the true time-frequency of 13:20. The recalibration of our Cosmic Time Travels through our **Galactic Purpose Signature** © (**GPS**) navigating Time Ship Earth through **2013**, to this present moment recounting the Lover's Script of Pascal Voton and Bolon Ik. We are coming full circle, and we, both man and woman, must HEAL ourselves to navigate safely into the new paradigm.

Queen Afua's call to action is a one-stop service station to tune up our temporary space suits so we can continue on our journey with a high quality of life into the new paradigm of light and love.

Brothers, our ancestors beseech us all to heed the call, and we will arise gracefully from our dynastic fall.

MAN HEAL THYSELF WELLNESS WARRIOR!

Asante Sana! Tua Neter! Medase Pa!

Baba Wanique Khemi~Tehuti Shabazz MD-NTS

Ambassador for Peace

Keeper of the Sacred Flame-Eagle

Director of Operations, WRFG 89.3 FM,

Atlanta CEO, Melanin 6 Corp.

www.waniqueshabazz.com

www.melanatedimmortals.com

JOURNEY OF POWERFUL PRACTICES

Khnum 'Stic' Ibomu

As one half of the hip-hop group dead prez, I am grateful to have toured the planet for decades, speaking our lyrical truth and reminding our communities that our collective political and social liberation is so much bigger than hip-hop. But even more than all of the political conversations, we have helped shift the impact far and wide, through spreading the vibes we first expressed in our song "Be Healthy." This significance has grown most dear to my heart.

The vision of creating the RBG FIT CLUB, the establishing of the fit-hop music category through the releases of my albums *The Workout* and *Workout II*, the development of becoming an avid runner, and the certification as a long-distance running coach are all manifestations of my healing as a result of beginning my healing journey with Queen Afua and her family.

Over twenty years ago, I woke up in extreme pain. The result being gout in my leg caused by a lifestyle of chronic stress, weed, alcohol abuse, and poor dietary habits. My wife Afya recommended that we apply the teachings and practices of Queen Afua to help me in restoring my health. Healing naturally from gout with Queen Afua's guidance put me on a path of holistic regeneration. My physical health, as well as my mental and spiritual health, became rejuvenated. Soon enough, I became aligned in my own path as a Wellness Warrior.

In the summer of 2001, I met SupaNova, Queen Afua's son, in Brooklyn at the International African Arts Festival. SupaNova's leadership as a Wellness Warrior hugely influenced the kind of artist I have grown into being. When I conceived and completed the Vegan Weightlifting Experiment, which became the book *Eat Plants, Lift Iron,* SupaNova's transformational example of plant-based bodybuilding offered an affirming inspiration.

The wealth of wellness wisdom that this Royal family exudes has profoundly impacted my life, my growth process, and my continued evolution. So, to say that I am very honored to share my thoughts would be a huge understatement. The affirmation "Man Heal Thyself" is our ancient inheritance. We healed ourselves since the beginning of existence by spending time with nature, observing natural cycles, eating and moving in tune with the natural ecosystem we are a part of. The natural lifestyle is the root and source of our regenerative powers. The more we align our actions with holistic principles of nature, the more we simultaneously and harmoniously empower ourselves.

As a result of my journey from gout to health, I became a Man. So, my understanding is that Health and Manhood are inseparable. All of the keys to wellness are also conveniently connected to Manhood. Within this book, *Man, Heal Thyself:*

The Wellness Warrior's Journey to Self-Mastery, Queen Afua and SupaNova give you a methodology that is invested in laying the bridge of Health and Manhood out before you in order to inspire your Greatness. Queen Afua and SupaNova are highly decorated Veterans of Wellness. They are Master Teachers of vitality and holistic practices. What Queen Afua and SupaNova have coordinated in this text is nothing short of a DIY manual for men's health and wellness.

May I encourage you to investigate, apply, and digest every bit! Use these practices and put in the work, not only to experience better health, but to acquire keys and assets of your own that will continue to benefit your life in numerous ways in the years to come.

STAY INSPIRED!

Khnum 'Stic' Ibomu
RBG FIT CLUB, Creative Director
Instagram: @Stic
RBGFITCLUB.com

THOUGHTS FROM THE EXAMINATION ROOM

Dr. Bernadette L. Sheridan

From the divine space of the Doctor's Exam Room, where men and women surrender pretense and ego to the desire to find answers, avoid pain, and prolong life, I join my voice with my fellow collaborators to repeat the timeliness of this work and the urgency of the situation.

I have been a practicing, traditionally trained, licensed, and Board Certified Family Practitioner for over thirty years. My entire career has been spent in two zip codes in Brooklyn, New York. The observations that I have made during that time are, no doubt, reflected in many other places around the country—rural, urban, upper class, and inner city. As a nation, we are becoming technologically advanced, but these impressive strides do not reflect a healthier population. In the 21st century, people still succumb to the same chronic illnesses as three decades ago, yet at much higher rates. Lack of access to care and information are minor reasons for the quantum leap to near epidemic numbers of hypertension, type 2 diabetes, heart disease, and cancer. People fill the clinics and offices in record numbers. At the same time, the Internet has made us all "research experts." Prescription drug sales account for billions of dollars in the Health Care Budget. Nonetheless, the statistics do not redeem us as a healthier population.

The last, chilling piece of the equation, the one that frosts the cake of urgency, is the fact that the children are now joining the ranks of the chronically ill, succumbing to "adult diseases" before they are even old enough to vote. We literally are dying to be well.

The solution, of course, is not found in a single place, but in a collaborative effort of things simple and things complex. There is no turning away from the fact that a toxic lifestyle based on consuming toxic food while growing up and growing old in a stressful century will require more and more pharmaceutical intervention to suppress its toxic effects. This book represents the first step to self-healing, and the simple realization that the car runs better and breaks down less if you fill it with quality fuel. It provides a template for healing, clear thinking, forgiveness, and release. Its message could not be timelier.

Kudos, thanks, and professional respect to Queen Afua, whom I have the privilege to know as a colleague and friend. From our first encounter, we recognized each other as healers on a common road. Because of that recognition and mutual respect, we have been able to blend our knowledge for a common good, proving that, yes, it is possible for holistic strategies and mainstream medicine to align. It is my hope and desire that her book finds a home in the consciousness of every man who reads it. To transform one ultimately has an effect on all. Respectfully submitted,

Bernadette L. Sheridan MD, F.A.A.F.P.
CEO, Grace Family Medical Practice
Brooklyn, New York

CHAPTER 10

WELLNESS WARRIORS & JUGGERNAUTS

THANK YOU, DOCTOR DAVIDSON

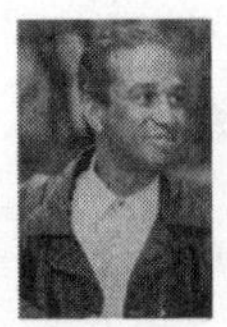

Dr. Ronald Davidson, a friend and colleague, a medical doctor, and a holistic physician, passed on into the ancestral realm in June 2006; he was 54 years young. Dr. Davidson fully absorbed the role of teaching the community to Heal Thyself. In his Brooklyn and Manhattan clinics, he had merged his allopathic and holistic practices decades before it became fashionable to do so. The fact that he never said "no" to any of us supported his decision to help us find the "yes" to our wellness. The entire community admired his laser-sharp mind and his hard work, as well as the bond he had with his patients. In the truest sense, as a profound man of medicine, he was a healing juggernaut . . . a Wellness Warrior.

It was Dr. Davidson who opened his doors to me to work in his clinic in the 1970s and 1980s, when I was but a neophyte in the Holistic Health field. Forgetting his own needs, he quickly and quietly moved from patient to patient to give them the best of his allopathic and holistic knowledge. Year in and year out, he took care of us. After writing a prescription for diabetic patients, he would insist they begin the exercise portion of their healing right then and there on the stationary bicycle in his clinic. Additionally, he understood the holistic importance of wellness brought by the cultural celebration of music and dance and artistic expression. Therefore, he set up "concerts" performed and attended by his patients. The concerts were healing for them and the community at large.

I worked with Dr. Davidson's patients, sharing my growing knowledge of holistic approaches to attain wellness for body, mind, and spirit. Although he wholeheartedly supported blending allopathic and holistic practices, at the time neither of us was financially prepared to launch a very costly clinical trial to prove the validity of East meets West for relief from illness and disease. For over two decades, I searched for the opportunity for the clinical trial to be born. Then I met Dr. Bernadette Sheridan. In 2009, she and I were able to conduct the clinical trial. Dr. Davidson would have been pleased.

REST IN POWER, DR. DAVIDSON. I DEDICATE TO YOU, THE DAY-TO-DAY LIFESTYLE OF MAN HEAL THYSELF.

Queen Afua

To The Healing Juggernaut Man, to all the men on your path to wellness, do not let the life and work of Dr. Davidson be in vain. In his honor and memory, pick up your shield and be encouraged to be a Heal Thyself Man valiantly on your journey to Optimal Wellness.

THE HEALING JUGGERNAUT MAN

We recognize and salute the Healing Juggernaut Man. You have been on the front line of wellness. You have been devoted to "the work" for over 10 years; some of you for over 30 and even 40 years. Be of courage; be inspired. All that you have contributed to raising the people has not gone in vain. Your healing hands have surrounded the world.

The Healing Juggernauts carried the natural medicine within them, as if it were in their loins, and shared their path of wellness with the multitude. First, they transformed themselves, and then they reached out to assist all others who were on a quest to take back their lives. The time has come, 2012 and beyond, where the masses are beginning to awaken and witness the wellness shift. The Businessman, the Cultural Man, the Spiritualist, the Health Activist Man have come for products and to workshops, seminars, and consultations, seeking wellness solutions. Now the Hustler Man and the brother from "Around the Way" Man are coming for wellness. They are "busting down the door." They want to get off the drugs, cigarettes, and alcohol that are poisoning their blood and stifling their thinking. They are seeking to stop the consumption of dead and infested flesh that's causing cancer and a short life expectancy. The Wellness Warrior Healing Juggernauts are pulling them onto the path of wellness.

The men have been crying out in silence for help to be saved, to be whole, and to overcome the life of toxicity, which is no life at all. The men who lack the knowledge of how to achieve wellness are coming to the Healing Juggernauts. They are seeking help to release themselves from the addictions that have chained them to their demise. The Juggernaut Man will help men come out of the dark alley. The Juggernaut Man will rescue the men who use over-the-counter drugs for temporary relief from toxic symptoms and who, when the effects of the drugs wear off, need more potent substances to numb the pain. Often these substances have been more over-the-counter drugs, illegal drugs, toxic food, and toxic sexual encounters. Still, the hurt didn't go away. The men have had enough and are ready to "take the monkey off their back."

The Holistic Medicine Men from the four directions, North, South, East, and West, walk in the footprints of the eldest ancestors to help the man in the midst of body, mind, spiritual, and relationship disparity. The Healing Juggernaut Men have stayed the course, held their ground, and paid their dues in order to be master healers. Be encouraged, Healing Juggernaut Man. We know for many it has been difficult to keep the faith. Remove your ego and continue to help the men who are bleeding now and have been for generations. Help them to break the chains that have destroyed lives in the form of poor dietary habits. Diseases of body, mind, and spirit have plagued generations from the days of plantation slavery to these new days of prison industrial slavery. Healing Juggernaut Man, we call upon you to help free the parents who conceive and birth sick babies. We look forward to the birth of well babies, who as returning giants can save humanity. The people have faith in the Healing Juggernaut Man.

Master Healers, Brothers, Fathers, Elders, Men in Wellness, you fought the system and you won. You stood for truth in the line of fire and did not bend. You held on tight for the people so that they could recover. You, the Healing Juggernaut, have walked the pathway and have become the living legacy of great, mighty, wise men. I feel profound gratitude for the spiritual architects, Wellness bricklayers, and holistic pyramid builders. You diligently worked the forces of nature as you packed, wrapped, smudged, sweated, and fed natural foods and herbs to the men and families in need. Through the laying on of hands and your prayers, you helped the seekers of Wellness. From the United States to the Caribbean, from the United Kingdom to Brazil and throughout the continent of Africa; to those I met face to face, and those I met in spirit, I thank you. Healing Juggernauts who carry knowledge and do the work, we appreciate you.

Queen Afua

MAN HEAL THYSELF JUGGERNAUTS

ARIT 1: THE FAMILY MAN OF UNITY AND WEALTH

"Finding a perfect model for your business passion will allow you to conduct business for years to come and create a legacy for those you choose to mentor."

ELLIS LIDDELL

ARIT 2: THE SENSUAL MAN OF HEIGHTENED SENSITIVITY

"Art is my saving grace; it is my center of power. I don't know who I would be or where I would be without art."

LEROY CAMPBELL

ARIT 3: THE TRANSFORMATION MAN OF RENEWAL

"A Healer is a person who is trained in and understands the elements that create healing of the people, the Earth, and the balance among all living beings."

JESSE R. BROWN, M.D.

ARIT 4: THE LOVER MAN OF HARMONY

"Be Proactive In Your Healing: When I say healing, I mean your mental, physical, and spiritual healing, because the issues in ourselves show up in so many ways."

CHRIS KAZI ROLLE

ARIT 5: THE COMMUNICATION MAN OF CONNECTIVITY AND CREATIVITY

"Queen Afua's call to action is a one-stop service station to tune up our temporary space suits so we can continue on our journey with a high quality of life into the new paradigm of light and love.

"Brothers, our ancestors beseech us all to heed the call, and we will arise gracefully from our dynastic fall."

WANIQUE SHABAZZ KHEMI-TEHUTI

ARIT 6: THE INTUITIVE MAN OF CLEAR VISION

"What is required of us men is to own up to the myths and misplaced motives we have about ourselves and our relationships. It is time to take responsibility for our behavior, which eventually has an impact not only on our lives, but also on the women and children in our lives."

LLOYD STRAYHORN

ARIT 7: THE UNIVERSAL HUMANITARIAN MAN

"If you tie it [healing] back to music, it is all very simple. If we all sing more every day and even drum or play any instrument, we will become more 'in tune' (pun intended) with the rhythm of life."

RAS KATRIEL WISE

ARIT 8: THE ILLUMINATED MAN OF ENLIGHTENMENT

"Brothers, your history has already paved the road for your future. Brothers, take ownership of your stories. Research who and where you come from to better understand where you are going and how you are going to get there. Make yourself timeless. The rest is history."

HRU KHUFU (ROBERT GAY)

ARIT 9: THE HARMONIZING MAN OF SERENITY

"To heal the planet, we must first heal ourselves. To heal ourselves, we must first know ourselves."

TAHARQA ALEEM

ARIT 10: THE NATURE MAN OF REGENERATION

"Although there is much necessary work to be done locally and nationally to eradicate food deserts and increase access for more people, eating good in the hood is doable. Healthy foods are mostly produce, which are the most simple and least expensive food options we have. Our eating habits are learned behaviors, and our taste buds can be reconditioned for healthy living. Place more value on life, and let's adopt healthier habits . . ."

STIC MAN IBOMU

ARIT 11: THE ALCHEMIST MAN OF CHANGE

"The accumulation of human wisdom from the most ancient civilization is a legacy . . . from pre–Nile Valley civilizations to the cutting edge of science-based, data-driven wisdom, we can bear witness to a vast spectrum of knowledge that can and does sustain health, prosperity, quality of human engagement, and sustained optimism about the future that lies ahead."

CHEF KEIDI AWADU

ARIT 12: THE SUPREME MAN OF SELF-MASTERY

"We are here to master the Being and to live it as humans . . . This academic brings a new consciousness; we are consciously and subconsciously illiterate to the greatness that is the true form of the self-identity. To heal the planet, we must heal our worlds. We must begin by going in on what makes us GOD!"

MEMNON UZAN

FINAL THOUGHTS

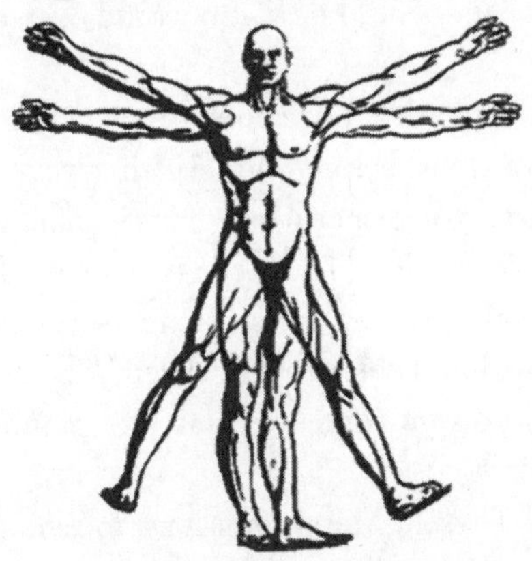

WORDS FROM MALCOLM X
(EL-HAJJ MALIK EL-SHABAZZ)

Daring to reach, to climb, to crawl, to scratch, to get back up when you've been knocked down, to push forward—ever forward—to forgive.
It means sacrificing everything if necessary, to carve out a place for your own existence.
It means living.

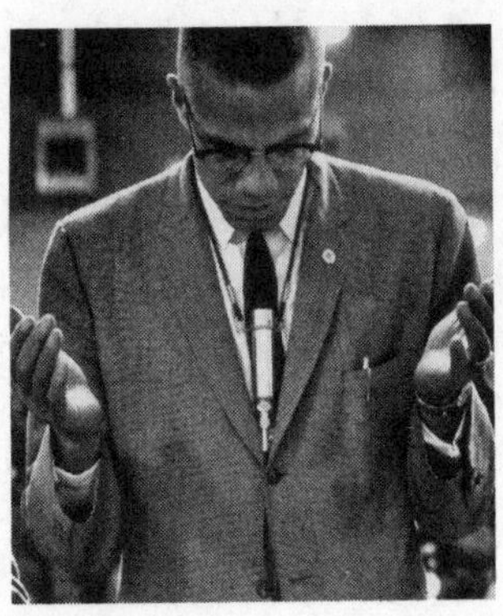

CHANGE

When you could not see yourself . . . beyond your imperfections and shortcomings, I saw you . . . your greatness . . . your radiant beauty . . . I knew you would overcome, make it happen . . .

Man, Heal Thyself. Your roots are your family members and those who came before you. All that you are has been passed down to you—sperm to ovum—man to woman—generation to generation. The seeds they planted yesterday—peace, war, wellness, madness, strife, serenity—represent their love denied and their love realized. Those seeds are in you. You are the sum total of what was planted into your bloodline.

Man, Heal Thyself. You do not have to remain a prisoner of the negative elements in your DNA, such as your mother's diabetes, father's prostate cancer, grandfather's Alzheimer's disease, or grandmother's fears. If you make changes to your lifestyle, you and your future bloodline can enjoy peace and Wellness. You can restore your Spiritual Wellness through prayer and meditation. You can detox from diseases and purify your physical anatomy by eating "live" foods, doing your bodywork, and striving to live a more holistic lifestyle. You can look at how you eat and how you live and decide what is working for you and what needs to be changed.

Man, pick up your bag and start walking on your 12-week journey to optimal wellness. With determination and commitment, you can rejuvenate your total being—physical, mental, spiritual, emotional, social, and even financial. You can overcome the negative DNA. As you holistically transform into a Heal Thyself Man, you will be planting new seeds for the next generations. Your life and the lives of your future family will be restored.

Many have gone before you, planting good seeds and doing good work.

Now it is your time. As a human, you have a birthright to wellness. As a Heal Thyself Man, you have a responsibility to make your wellness happen. Make that change.

QUEEN AFUA

ACKNOWLEDGMENTS

I am grateful for uncountable blessings from on High.

It is my honor to acknowledge SupaNova for his dedication and commitment to Stand in the Gap for the men who gather from the four directions to Heal Themselves. To Halleluyah Walcott for shouldering SupaNova Slom as they stand in unison to RESTORE Our Brothers in Body, Mind, and Spirit.

To the Ancestors: I acknowledge all the ancestral Holistic Healing Men whose shoulders I stand upon to continue the Wellness Work. Special gratitude to Wellness Warriors: Imhotep of the Nile Valley, Father of Ancient and Modern Medicine.

I am grateful for beloved elders, activists, entrepreneurs, and inspirations; each in your own way, Wellness Warriors. I give thanks to Baaba Heru Ankh Ra Semahj Se Ptah (The Studio of Ptah) for masterfully teaching the wisdom of the Nile Valley Legacy.

A particular appreciation to the 12 Healing Juggernauts for the Man Heal Thyself Empowerment Circle. Their work to raise up our men from out of the depths of despair, alcohol, and all challenges, to heal and to show up for their family in a more balanced way. They work toward guiding men to take their health seriously as they nurture themselves to well-being.

- ★ Ellis Lidell—The Family Man of Unity and Wealth
- ★ Leroy Campbell—The Sensual Artistic Man of Heightened Sensitivity
- ★ Dr. Jesse Brown—The Holistic Transformative Man of Renewal
- ★ Chris Kazi Rolle—The Lover Man of Harmony
- ★ Wanique Shabazz Khemi-Tehuti—The Communication Man of Connectivity and Creativity
- ★ Lloyd Strayhorn—The Intuitive Man of Clear Vision
- ★ Ras Katriel Wise—The Universal Humanitarian Man of Global Wellness
- ★ Seed HRU KHUPU (Robert Gay)—The Illuminated Man
- ★ Taharqa Aleem—The Harmonizing Man of Serenity
- ★ stic.man Ibomu—The Nature Man of Regeneration
- ★ Chef Keidi Awadu—The Alchemist Man of Change
- ★ Memnon Uzan—The Supreme Man of Optimal Wellness

Thank you . . .

REFERENCE AND CITATION SOURCES

Albertine, Kurt H., *Anatomica's Body Atlas*, Thunder Bay Press, 2006

Alexander, Michelle. *The New Jim Crow: Mass Incarceration in the Age of Colorblindness.* New York: New Press, 2010.

American Heart Association, Heart Disease and Stroke Statistics: A Report from the 2010 National Survey on Drug Use and Health. September 2010. Web. 21 December 2011.

American Lung Association, Epidemiology and Statistics Unit, *Trends in Lung Cancer Morbidity and Mortality.* November 2014.

Balch, Phyliss A., *Prescription for Herbal Healing*, Avery Trade, 2002

Balch, Phyliss A., and James F. Balch, *Prescription for Nutritional Healing*, Avery Trade, 2010.

Budge, E. A. Wallis, *The Papyrus of Ani (The Egyptian Book of The Dead)*, New York: Putnam, 1913.

Centers for Disease Control and Prevention, "Arthritis-Related Statistics," 18 July 2018, Accessed 9 February 2021. www.cdc .gov/arthritis/data_statistics/arthritisrelated-stats.htm.

Dale, Cyndi, *The Subtle Body: An Encyclopedia of Your Energetic Anatomy*, Sounds True Adult, 2009.

Gerber, Richard. *Practical Guide to Vibrational Medicine: Energy Healing & Spiritual Transformation*, New York: HarperCollins, 2001.

Jack, Leonard. "Diabetes and Men's Health Issues." *Diabetes*

Spectrum, 17, no. 4 (1 Oct. 2004), pp. 206–208, spectrum.diabetesjournals.org/content/17/4/206.full,10.2337/diaspect.17.4.206. Accessed 10 Feb. 2021.

Leigh, J. Adam, et al. "Ethnic Minorities and Coronary Heart Disease: An Update and Future Directions." *Current Atherosclerosis Reports*, 18, no. 2 (20 Jan. 2016), www.ncbi.nlm.nih.gov/pmc/articles/PMC4828242/, 10.1007/s11883-016-0559-4.

Noecker, MD, Robert J. "How to Treat Glaucoma: Surgery, Causes, Symptoms & Prevention." *EMedicineHealth*, (25 May 2020), www.emedicinehealth.com/glaucoma_overview/article_em.htm. Accessed 10 Feb. 2021.

Souls of Black Men: African American Men Discuss Mental Health, Community Voices, Satcher Health Leadership Institute of Morehouse School of Medicine. 21 July 2003, Web: 21 December 2011.

Stone, Robin D., *No Secrets No Lies: How Black Families Can Heal from Sexual Abuse*, Broadway, 2004.

Substance Abuse and Mental Health Services Administration. (2011). "Results from the 2010 National Survey on Drug Use and Health: Volume I. Summary of National Findings" Web: 6 Jan. 2012.

Udo, Erasmus. *Fats That Heal, Fats That Kill: The Complete Guide to Fats, Oils, Cholesterol and Human Health*, Alive Books, 1993.

Woods, V. Diane, Susanne B. Montgomery, Juan Carlos Belliard, et al., "Culture, Black Men, and Prostate Cancer: What Is Reality?" *Cancer Control*, 11, no. 6 (2004 Nov.-Dec.): 388–396, www.medscape.com/viewarticle/497924. Accessed 9 Feb. 2021.

ABOUT THE AUTHOR

SupaNova Slom is a multifaceted artist, musician, holistic healer, and wellness coach renowned for his contributions to the hip-hop community and his advocacy for holistic health and wellness. As the son of Queen Afua, a celebrated holistic health practitioner and author, he has been deeply influenced by principles of wellness and consciousness.

Throughout his career in the music industry as a rapper and producer, SupaNova Slom has consistently woven themes of health, wellness, and consciousness into his music. He is the author of *The Remedy: The Five-Week Power Plan to Detox Your System, Combat the Fat, and Rebuild Your Mind and Body*, a book that emphasizes detoxification and holistic health principles.

SupaNova Slom's commitment to wellness is further demonstrated through his involvement in the "Man Heal Thyself" program, based on the best-selling book he co-authored with his mother, Queen Afua, *Man, Heal Thyself*. In both the book and the program, they encourage men to take charge of their physical, mental, and spiritual health through holistic healing practices, offering wellness protocols to strengthen social, emotional, and spiritual wellness on the journey to self-mastery.